ESSENTIAL RESEARCH FINDINGS

IN CHILD AND ADOLESCENT COUNSELLING AND PSYCHOTHERAPY

PRAISE FOR THE BOOK

'This book is the "go-to" resource for all those involved in supporting young people.'
Dr Andrew Reeves, Chair, British Association for Counselling and Psychotherapy

'This is a ground breaking book for counsellors and psychotherapists working with children and young people. The contributors acknowledge the scepticism of many practitioners in relation to adopting an "evidence based approach," and each chapter is likely to provoke debate and discussion. For me the power of this book lies in the way the authors employ their own self-reflexivity to model an approach to evidence-based practice, and suggest ways their readers might set about finding and examining evidence themselves. Through reading this work, each of us may, indeed, become "research-invigorated."'
Professor Miranda Wolpert, Director of the Evidence Based Practice Unit (UCL and the Anna Freud National Centre for Children and Families) and of Child Outcomes Research Consortium

'*Essential Research Findings in Child and Adolescent Counselling and Psychotherapy* makes an invaluable contribution to research-informed practice with younger clients. Written by some of the leading figures in the field, it provides practitioners with an authoritative and accessible overview of up-to-date scientific knowledge.'
John McLeod, University of Oslo

'With contributions from a range of experts, the text offers specific therapeutic guidance for working effectively with children and young people with mental health problems, drawing on the latest research evidence.'
Panos Vostanis, Professor of Child Mental Health, University of Leicester; Visiting Professor, University College London; Editor of *British Counselling and Psychotherapy Research*

'There are two strongly held narratives around today about what makes for a good counsellor or psychotherapist: the narrative of "clinical experience" verses the narrative of "research evidence". This book skilfully brings these two narratives together into a coherent and complementary whole. It provides an engaging overview of research in the field of children and young people's psychological therapies written by some of the world leaders in the field. It is not a book about research but more helpfully, it is a book about how to understand and use research evidence, to blend with clinical experience, to become a better therapist. It is one of the most accessible and comprehensive summaries of the research evidence that I have read – essential for all who are serious about their therapeutic practice.'
Duncan Law is a Consultant Clinical Associate at the Anna Freud National Centre for Children and Young People, an Honorary Senior Lecturer at University College London and Director of MindMonkey Associates

ESSENTIAL RESEARCH FINDINGS

in CHILD and ADOLESCENT
COUNSELLING and PSYCHOTHERAPY

EDITED BY

NICK MIDGLEY ✱ **JACQUELINE HAYES** ✱ **MICK COOPER**

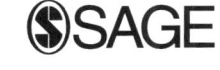

Los Angeles | London | New Delhi
Singapore | Washington DC | Melbourne

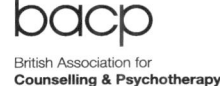

British Association for
Counselling & Psychotherapy

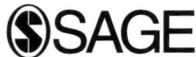

Los Angeles | London | New Delhi
Singapore | Washington DC | Melbourne

SAGE Publications Ltd
1 Oliver's Yard
55 City Road
London EC1Y 1SP

SAGE Publications Inc.
2455 Teller Road
Thousand Oaks, California 91320

SAGE Publications India Pvt Ltd
B 1/I 1 Mohan Cooperative Industrial Area
Mathura Road
New Delhi 110 044

SAGE Publications Asia-Pacific Pte Ltd
3 Church Street
#10-04 Samsung Hub
Singapore 049483

Editor: Susannah Trefgarne
Editorial assistant: Edward Coats
Production editor: Rachel Burrows
Copyeditor: Jane Fricker
Proofreader: Brian McDowell
Indexer: Adam Pozner
Marketing manager: Camille Richmond
Cover design: Lisa Harper-Wells
Typeset by: C&M Digitals (P) Ltd, Chennai, India
Printed in the UK

Library of Congress Control Number: 2016961868

British Library Cataloguing in Publication data

A catalogue record for this book is available from
the British Library.

ISBN 978-1-4129-6249-0
ISBN 978-1-4129-6250-6 (pbk)

Jac would like to dedicate her two chapters (Chapter 6 and Chapter 7) to her mum:

To Stella Hayes (1954–2015), with so much love, and thanks, for giving me life. X

CONTENTS

ABOUT THE EDITORS AND CONTRIBUTORS

Nick Midgley is a child and adolescent psychotherapist at the Anna Freud National Centre for Children and Families, and a Senior Lecturer in the Research Department of Clinical, Educational and Health Psychology at University College London, where he is co-director of the Child Attachment and Psychological Therapies Research Unit (ChAPTRe). His publications include *Child psychotherapy and research: New directions, emerging findings* (Routledge, 2009) and *Minding the child: Mentalization-based interventions with children, young people and families* (Routledge, 2013).

Jacqueline Hayes works as a Lecturer in Counselling Psychology at the University of Roehampton. In therapeutic practice, she works with adults and young people, and has a special practice interest in working psychologically with hearing voices. Previously she has worked at the Anna Freud Centre and the University of Manchester.

Mick Cooper is a Professor of Counselling Psychology at the University of Roehampton and a chartered psychologist. Mick is author and editor of a range of texts on person-centred, existential and relational approaches to therapy, including *Existential therapies* (2nd ed., Sage, 2017), *Working at relational depth in counselling and psychotherapy* (Sage, 2005, with Dave Mearns) and *Pluralistic counselling and psychotherapy* (Sage, 2011, with John McLeod). Mick has also led a range of research studies exploring the process and outcomes of humanistic counselling with young people.

Elizabeth Allison is the Director of the Psychoanalysis Unit in the Research Department of Clinical, Educational and Health Psychology at University College London. She is a psychoanalyst and Member of the British Psychoanalytical Society. With Peter Fonagy and Mary Target she is Editor of Karnac's Developments in Psychoanalysis book series. She holds a doctorate in English Literature from the University of Oxford.

Clare Brunst works as a researcher at an early detection service for psychosis in East London NHS Foundation Trust. Previously, she worked on research projects at the Anna Freud Centre and the University of Ottawa. She has also worked therapeutically with children and adolescents with special education needs in schools.

Peter Fonagy is Freud Memorial Professor of Psychoanalysis and Head of the Research Department of Clinical, Educational and Health Psychology at University College London; Chief Executive of the Anna Freud National Centre for Children and Families, London; Consultant to the Child and Family Program at the Menninger Department of Psychiatry and Behavioral Sciences at Baylor College of Medicine, Houston; and holds visiting professorships at Yale and Harvard Medical Schools.

Ann Hagell is Research Lead at the Association for Young People's Health (AYPH) in London. She is a chartered psychologist and has published widely on topics relating to young people's wellbeing. Ann has worked with a range of universities, think-tanks and funders over the past 25 years and is committed to making research findings relevant and useful to policy and practice. She is Consulting Editor of the *Journal of Adolescence*, and prior to working with AYPH she ran the Changing Adolescence programme at the Nuffield Foundation (2006–2012). She is also a professional advisor to the Research in Practice Partnership Board.

Terry Hanley is the Programme Director for the Doctorate in Counselling Psychology at the University of Manchester. He is a Fellow of the Higher Education Academy, an Associate Fellow of the British Psychological Society and was Editor of *Counselling Psychology Review* between the years 2009 and 2015. He has a keen interest in training therapists in research skills and is a co-author of *Introducing counselling and psychotherapy research* (Sage, 2012). Additionally, his own therapeutic practice and research has primarily focused around work with young people and young adults, a topic on which he is also lead editor of the text *Adolescent counselling psychology* (Routledge, 2012).

Barbara Maughan is Professor of Developmental Epidemiology at the MRC Social, Genetic and Developmental Psychiatry Centre, Institute of Psychiatry, Psychology and Neuroscience, King's College London. After a short period in social work she moved into research, and has been researching aspects of child mental health problems for much of her career. Her work has spanned epidemiological studies of childhood disorders; early risk factors for childhood difficulties; and the long-term implications of mental health problems in childhood for health and wellbeing in adult life. She has also investigated historical trends in rates of childhood emotional and behavioural difficulties, and wider societal factors that may contribute to variations in children's vulnerability over time.

Graham Music is a consultant child and adolescent psychotherapist at the Tavistock and Portman Clinics and an adult psychotherapist in private practice. His publications include *Nurturing natures* (2nd ed., Psychology Press, 2016), *Affect and emotion* (Icon Books, 2001), and *The good life* (Routledge, 2014). Formerly Associate Clinical Director of the Tavistock's child and family department, he has managed a range of services working with child maltreatment and neglect. He currently works clinically with forensic cases at the Portman Clinic. He teaches, lectures and supervises on a range of training programmes in Britain and abroad.

Julia Noble is a counselling psychologist based in Manchester, having previously working in Cambridge on psychological test development for children and adults.

She has a strong interest in working alongside young people, having worked therapeutically in children's services and higher educational establishments.

Alana Ryan is a research and policy officer in the Research Department of Clinical, Educational and Health Psychology, University College London. She holds an MSc in Comparative Social Policy from the University of Oxford and a BA in Philosophy, Political Science, Economics and Sociology from Trinity College Dublin.

ACKNOWLEDGEMENTS

This project was supported by funding from the British Association for Counselling and Psychotherapy (BACP). We would like to thank Nancy Rowland, Andy Hill, Angela Couchman, and colleagues at the BACP for all their help and encouragement in bringing the book to fruition.

Thanks to Susannah Trefgarne, Rachel Burrows, Edward Coats, and the other members of the Sage Publications team for their enthusiasm about the project, and all their hard work in getting us through from the original idea to the present text.

We would like to extend a special thank you to Clare Brunst and Fiona Robinson for their help in supporting the process of putting this book together. Thanks also to Teresa Robertson and Lawrence Dodgson, whose illustrations bring the ideas in Chapter 3 alive so well; and to Michelle Sleed and the PsychD students at Anna Freud/UCL for their contribution to the research glossary.

Some sections of Chapter 1 are reprinted, with permission, from the following two journal articles by Nick Midgley: 'Sailing between Scylla and Charybdis: Incorporating qualitative approaches into child psychotherapy research', published by Taylor and Francis in the *Journal of Child Psychotherapy* (© Association of Child Psychotherapists); and 'Disseminators vs. revisionists: Attitudes to the implementation gap in evidence based practice', published by Emerald Group Publishing Ltd in the *Journal of Children's Services*.

Nick would like to thank his colleagues and students at UCL and the Anna Freud National Centre for Children and Families; and Kiriko and Thomas, for their continuing support and inspiration.

Jac would like to say a special thank you to her Dad, and to Jo and Lou.

Mick would like to thank colleagues at the Centre for Research in Social and Psychological Transformation (CREST) at the University of Roehampton; and Maya, Ruby, Shula and Zac.

1

INTRODUCTION: WHAT CAN CHILD THERAPISTS LEARN FROM RESEARCH?

NICK MIDGLEY, JACQUELINE HAYES AND MICK COOPER

This chapter discusses

- The rationale for integrating research evidence into therapeutic work with children and young people
- The emergence of the concept of 'evidence-based practice'
- The limits of research evidence
- The value of research evidence
- The aims of this book
- The format of this book and its chapters
- Our reflections, as co-editors, on the stances we bring to this book

Talia sits in her chair staring blankly at her therapist. It's the start of the second session. Talia is 14, and has been referred to therapy because she's missing school, unable to concentrate in class, and getting into fights with her parents. Talia's therapist can feel her anger and resentment bubbling underneath the surface. In the first session of therapy, Talia talked about how she hates her mum now, how things at home are 'rubbish' and that she doesn't get to do what she wants because she's always looking after her little brother. It's been like that, she says, since her nan died. The first session seemed to go ok: Talia told her therapist a bit about what's been happening and set some goals for the therapy work, including that she wanted to be able to get on better with her mum. But now, sitting opposite Talia who stares blankly into space, the therapist is wondering what to do next, and how to help Talia find some way of expressing herself and getting the support and help she needs.

What can reading a book about research findings offer to the woman sitting with Talia, when trying to help her work effectively as a child therapist? Traditionally, most counsellors and psychotherapists would probably have said, 'Not much'. In an interesting study of the 'Utilization of psychotherapy research by practicing psychotherapists', Morrow-Bradley and Elliott (1986) found that the typical psychotherapist does not find research studies useful to practice. The psychotherapists said that they didn't feel that the variables selected in most research studies reflected actual clinical practice; data analyses overemphasized group statistics and statistical significance against the particularity of the clinical encounter; research findings were not translated into a clinically useful format; and they often lacked the suitable training, or were simply too busy, to read research papers. Consistent with this, when counsellors and psychotherapists are asked in what ways they learn most about their work, studies have consistently found that 'research' is bottom of the list – below clinical experience, supervision, personal therapy, case presentations and discussion with colleagues.

So what is the reason for this research–practice gap? In another interesting study, Darlington and Scott (2002) found that psychotherapists associated the word 'research' with such terms as 'hard', 'cold', 'scientific', 'factual', 'time-consuming' and 'tedious'. By contrast, the same participants associated the word 'practice' with such terms as 'subjective', 'people', 'messy', 'soft', 'warm', 'flexible' – clearly, a more positive set of associations.

Despite these findings, this book aims to make the case that therapeutic work with children and young people can benefit from an engagement with the research evidence. As we will elaborate on later in this introduction, this does not mean that research evidence should be treated like some form of deity that we all need to worship (Cooper, 2008). Other sources of inspiration – such as clinical experience, supervision, personal therapy, case presentations, discussion with colleagues – can all have enormous value. But research evidence is one source of knowledge frequently overlooked by therapists, and we think it is an essential one. Still, today, we train practitioners in all sorts of different practices with children and young people without knowing enough about what the research findings can tell us. Too much theory and not enough evidence: the aim of this book is to try and redress the balance. So that, when we are sitting there with a young person like Talia, we can draw from our training, and we can draw from our theoretical knowledge, and our experience as therapists, but we can also draw from the research findings – a treasure trove of knowledge that is just waiting to be unlocked.

The birth of evidence-based practice

Since Morrow-Bradley and Elliott (1986) surveyed therapists in 1985, there has been an increasing focus on engaging with, and drawing on, empirical research – often promoted under the umbrella term 'evidence-based practice' (EBP). This can be defined as 'the conscientious, explicit and judicious use of current best evidence in decision making about the care of individual patients' (Sackett, Rosenberg, Muir Gray, Haynes, & Richardson, 1996: 71). In practice, this means integrating individual clinical expertise with the best available external evidence from systematic research.

If there is one person who is probably responsible for the concept of EBP, it is a Professor of Tuberculosis and Chest Diseases called Archie Cochrane. In 1972 Cochrane wrote a book called *Effectiveness and efficiency: Random reflections on health services*. In it, he made a powerful attack on the medical establishment of his day, in which he argued that 'chaotic, individualistic, often ineffective and sometimes harmful' patterns of care were the norm, largely due to the fact that medicine itself had not organized its knowledge 'in any systematic, reliable and cumulative way' (quoted in Oakley, Gough, Oliver, & Thomas, 2005: 5]. In its place, he wrote, doctors should establish a system of 'evidence-based medicine', in which evidence for the effectiveness of medical interventions should be systematically assessed and form the basis for treatment choices. Cochrane's book was initially targeted at the field of medicine, but his simple message, about the inevitable limitation of resources and the importance of using evidence from research to establish which approaches are most effective, quickly caught on. His work led to the opening of the first Cochrane Centre in 1992 and the founding of the Cochrane Collaboration (www.cochranecollaboration.com) in 1993. By then his ideas were influential across the whole field of social care and mental health; and the impact of his ideas has continued to broaden out even further in the last 25 years to cover almost every aspect of public life.

While Cochrane's ideas have been hugely influential, what is less well-known is why he first developed these ideas. In his autobiography, Cochrane describes how, as a young medical officer, he was captured by the German army, and found himself in a prisoner of war camp in the early 1940s, caring for a motley group of prisoners of various nationalities, many of whom were suffering from tuberculosis. Cochrane and his colleagues attended to the men as best as they could, herded together behind a wire fence. However many of the soldiers whom he cared for, and came to think of as friends, did not survive, and Cochrane found himself taking the role of priest as much as physician. Looking back many years later, Cochrane remembered a day when he found a propaganda pamphlet which had been dropped inside the camp, championing the 'clinical freedom and democracy' that would be achieved if the Allies were to win the war. Recalling this experience, Cochrane wrote:

> I found it impossible to understand. I had considerable freedom of clinical choice of therapy: my trouble was that I did not know which to use and when. I would gladly have sacrificed my freedom for a little knowledge. I had never heard then of 'randomized controlled trials', but I knew there was no real evidence that anything we had to offer had any effect on tuberculosis, and I was afraid that I shortened the lives of some of my friends by unnecessary intervention. (Cochrane, 1972: 6)

This uncertainty about the knowledge-base for his medical practice stayed with Cochrane after the war, and resulted many years later in the publication of his book on evidence-based medicine. Cochrane never wanted doctors to face the situation he had himself faced as a young man, in which he risked shortening his patients' lives because of his lack of knowledge about appropriate methods of treatment. If evidence could be accumulated from lots of doctors, about lots of treatments for lots of patients, perhaps this body of knowledge could be used to improve the chances for patients – or at least it might make his decision-making better informed than he had been when relying only on the trials and errors of his own medical career.

The limitations of research

Of course, there are many good reasons why child therapists should be wary of research findings (Cooper, 2008). For a start, research talks mostly in generalities rather than specifics. So, for instance, a research study might show that depressed clients, on average, will improve with cognitive behavioural therapy, but this does not mean that a specific individual, such as Talia, will find benefit in this approach. The probability is that she will, but she may not, and it is also possible that she will feel a lot worse after it. In this respect, to base therapeutic practice wholly on empirical research findings – to the exclusion of other factors, such as the expressed preference of the young person – would be profoundly unethical. Counselling and psychotherapy research findings can only ever tell us about what is most likely to happen – they cannot give us certainties.

Then there is the problem that research findings cannot fully capture the complexity of what happens in the therapeutic process. They are necessarily reductionist and approximate. An outcome measure is, after all, a standardized questionnaire that tries to capture change in a numerical way, but it cannot tell us the meaning of that number. Talia, for example, two sessions in, may actually report feeling sadder and more tearful than when she started therapy, because she is starting to realize that behind her anger, she really misses her nan. This may make her score on an outcome measure look the same as when she started, or perhaps even worse. Does this mean the therapy is not working? Not necessarily. And it may also be, for instance, that Talia is having fewer arguments with her mum, but the form she is filling out does not ask her much about this, and so there is no box to tick. And when she is asked to fill out a different form, this time about something called the 'alliance', her score is in the moderate range, suggesting that her relationship with her therapist is neither strong nor weak. But, again, this does not capture the reality: that sometimes Talia feels so close to her therapist that it is just like talking to her nan again; but then, when her therapist is too 'bossy', she just reminds her of her mum and Talia just wants to get out of there.

Another limitation of research findings is that they will inevitably be influenced by the researchers' own assumptions and biases. That is, even when research is conducted in a highly rigorous way, biases still manage to creep in. From the research question or topic, to the methods employed, to the way findings are written up, choices are being made by people (researchers) who live and work in a particular social, cultural and political climate. This means that we should always read research findings in a critical way, paying attention to the background and context of who conducted the research and what their agendas might be.

Research findings are also always arrived at through the use of some particular tool, measure or procedure, and these will inevitably influence the kinds of findings that are reported. (Indeed, even the word 'findings' suggests that what the researchers report was just sitting there, waiting to be 'found', rather than the reality that is that evidence is always constructed, at least to some degree, by the way the research team has framed their investigations.) If psychological wellbeing is defined and measured in terms of an absence of mental illness, for instance, the kinds of therapies that are shown to be most effective may be different to those where it is defined and measured in terms of a potential for growth. Researchers can even come up with radically different conclusions from the same set of data if they use different tools of analysis. It is also important to bear in mind that research is always conducted with a particular sample of people, such that the generalizability of its findings will always be limited.

Even if it were possible for researchers and research tools to be entirely objective, value-free and comprehensive, we are still faced with the fact that the scientific method, itself, is not an assumption-free tool, but a particular way of understanding the world that is based on a specific set of assumptions (for instance, that events in the world are linked together by cause-and-effect relationships). So while, within the scientific framework, it may be possible to prove or disprove that certain things are true (though even that is questionable), it is never possible to prove that science, itself, is the 'truest' way of understanding the world.

Another reason why therapists can be critical of evidence-based practice is because it can be experienced as a devaluing of professional competence, insofar as it can lead to assertions that 'young people presenting with X should be offered Y because the evidence-based guidelines say so'. When coupled with decision-making by commissioners of a similar sort (i.e. 'We won't commission X because the guidelines say that Y is the best treatment for Z'), it is not surprising that evidence-based practice often meets significant resistance in the workplace, where it is sometimes regarded as an inflexible system that over-rides the important local contexts in which decisions are made in response to complex situations. At its worst, there is a danger that evidence-based practice may lead to a rigid, unthinking system that works against the very aims that it strives for – to improve outcomes and the quality of care. The gap between research and practice – between evidence-based practice and evidence-based practitioners – is at risk of being maintained.

The value of research

Research findings, then, are by no means an infallible guide to practice, but they can still be of enormous help in day-to-day clinical practice (Cooper, 2008). For a start, they can give therapists some very good ideas about where to start from in the absence of other information. Research can only ever tell us about the likelihood of certain things happening, but that knowledge can be enormously valuable when integrated with other sources of knowledge to inform our decision-making.

So, for instance, Talia's therapist may find it very helpful to think about the way in which this young woman relates to her and others in terms of 'attachment', and whether Talia's somewhat 'dismissive' pattern of relating is associated with her early experiences of care-giving. As discussed in Chapter 3, attachment research, along with research in early parent–child interaction, can give a helpful framework to make sense of how a child or young person has come to experience difficulties. Similarly, research on the process and outcomes of therapy can function as a very helpful guide to practice. So, with Talia, it could be useful to know that both sadness and anger are typical features of depression in adolescence, and to be able to draw on guidelines that indicate which kinds of therapy have been most successful with young people suffering from depression. Or, at a more micro level, it may be helpful to find out what research suggests about specific therapeutic techniques. For example, Talia's therapist may benefit from knowing that research studies have suggested that problem-solving techniques are generally helpful with depression, but that it is essential to establish a good therapeutic relationship before launching into tasks and techniques. She may also find it helpful to know that this relationship is best built by a child or young person having control over the pace of therapy. This is not to say that those research findings will necessarily apply in Talia's case. Her therapist may discover that Talia actually dislikes problem-solving techniques, but until the therapist has a clear sense of what that particular young person wants or needs, the research evidence can provide a valuable source of guidance on what might be useful.

Research findings can also be very helpful in encouraging us to critically reconsider our assumptions about what works and does not work in therapy. For instance, we may assume that the best way to help Talia is to focus on her and get her to talk about herself rather than other people. But, as will be discussed in Chapter 6, there is evidence that giving young people time to talk about their relationships with their families can be more helpful than a solely 'internal' focus. This does not mean that asking Talia questions about herself are going to be unhelpful, but it may make us think about whether to balance our questions about Talia with some enquiry about the other important people in her life. In this respect, research findings can help us be more open to the myriad ways in which children and young people may be helped in therapy. At best, research can broaden our ways of thinking, introduce new perspectives, and encourage us to adhere less rigidly to one particular set of choices.

Within the world of contemporary healthcare practices, there is another very good reason, albeit a more pragmatic one, why child therapists should be aware of the research findings: to communicate to others about their work, and to help families (and commissioners of services) understand the value of what it is that they do. Today, it is rarely enough to say to a commissioning agency, 'I really think you should employ me because *I* know that what I do is helpful.' And why should it be? Funding bodies, whether large-scale organizations or private individuals, are becoming increasingly critical consumers, and want concrete evidence with which to justify their expenditures. So with so much high-quality evidence demonstrating the value that therapy can have, it would seem entirely self-defeating for therapists not to have a good working knowledge of this evidence. As the research itself shows, counsellors and psychotherapists tend to underestimate the strong research support for certain positive therapy findings (Boisvert & Faust, 2006), so knowing what the research really says can help therapists feel more confident in promoting their work.

Developing this book

Given these arguments, this book is written from the perspective that research is an invaluable component in the training of therapists for children and young people, and that it is important for us all to develop a level of *research literacy* in our everyday practice. By 'research literacy', we mean both the capacity to read and understand research studies, but also to be able to evaluate them critically, to understand their limitations as well as their strengths, and to make use of their findings in a judicious way. Such literacy is not straightforward, especially when much research is written in an impenetrable academic style that often makes it hard for the lay-reader to follow the points being made. Furthermore, the sheer amount of research being published month-by-month makes it almost impossible for busy therapists to keep up with the latest findings, or to be aware of any but the most high-profile studies.

It was with these issues in mind that we decided to put together this book. While recognizing the impossibility of being entirely comprehensive, we wanted to ask experts in their fields to try and bring together the key research findings in their area, summarized in a form that would make sense to therapists working with children and young people, and making clear what the potential significance of these findings might be for our practice. The basic template for this book was Mick's *Essential research findings in counselling and psychotherapy: The facts are friendly* (Sage, 2008), which strove to achieve something similar in the adult therapy field. As with Mick's original text, although our focus is on the findings themselves, we hope this book can also help to de-mystify the process of research itself, both by providing explanations of key research terms and giving examples of how particular studies came to the conclusions they reached.

The position we have taken in this book is explicitly pluralistic, in two particular respects. First, it is pluralistic in regard to the kinds of research that we believe are of relevance to child counsellors and therapists. There is a danger that the term 'research' can sometimes be used too narrowly to refer only to outcome research, or research evaluating the effectiveness of a particular type of therapy. Although we have included chapters on such research in this book, we believe that there is a much broader range of research that is relevant to clinical practice. For instance, we have chapters that review key findings from epidemiological research, as well as developmental and neuroscientific research, and research examining the process of psychotherapy.

Our approach is also pluralistic in regard to the types of research methodologies that have been used in the studies that are discussed. Rather than thinking in terms of a hierarchy of evidence, in which randomized controlled trials are better than, for example, qualitative research studies (see Chapter 4), we believe that different questions can be best answered by using different research designs. The chapters in this book therefore draw on a wide range of research methodologies and, partly for that reason, they may sometimes reach somewhat different conclusions. As a reader, this has the potential to be confusing, but it is the nature of research, and an important reason why we need to be both cautious and critical in the way we interpret research findings. No research findings are 'objectively' true, and for each study we must ask ourselves how it came to the conclusions it reached, and to what degree those conclusions may carry over into other contexts.

Overview

This book has six main chapters. Following this introduction, Ann Hagell and Barbara Maughan look at the epidemiology of child mental health (Chapter 2), i.e. the extent to which children and adolescents experience mental health problems, and the various factors associated with higher levels of distress. Chapter 3, by Graham Music, then looks at some of the key developmental factors that can cause mental health problems in children and young people, with a particular focus on neurobiological and attachment-related processes. Chapter 4, by Terry Hanley and Julia Noble, reviews the evidence for the effectiveness of counselling and psychotherapy with children and young people, overall. This is then broken down in more detail in Chapter 5, by Peter Fonagy, Liz Allison and Alana Ryan, who focus on the specific types of therapy that have been found to lead to positive therapeutic outcomes for children and young people with a range of specific psychiatric diagnoses. In Chapter 6, by Jacqueline Hayes, this exploration is developed further, by looking at the other factors – such as the quality of the therapeutic alliance – that are associated with positive therapeutic outcomes. Finally, Chapter 7, by Jacqueline Hayes and Clare Brunst, looks specifically at the evidence for particular techniques and practices in therapy with children and young people. The last chapter of the book, our Conclusion (Chapter 8), aims to draw the research findings together. Finally, we present a Glossary to help define and clarify the research terms used throughout this text, which we hope child therapists will also find useful when reading other research papers.

Although this book aims to give an overview of research findings in therapy with children and young people, there are inevitably gaps and omissions. For example, Graham Music's review of the developmental research in Chapter 3 does not cover all aspects of child development (for instance, cognitive development), as this would be a book (or a series of books) in itself. His chapter focuses primarily on neuroscience, genetics and attachment research, as areas with great potential to inform therapeutic work with children. Likewise, as most outcome research has been organized around specific psychiatric diagnoses, Fonagy et al.'s chapter does not review evidence for problems that fall outside of specific diagnostic categories (for instance, bullying). Furthermore, the research in all of these fields is developing rapidly and, even as these chapters are being written, new research findings are being published that may revise what has been written. In our concluding chapter, we discuss some of the ways in which therapists working with children and young people can try to keep themselves updated with key research findings – without having to give up their day-job and spend the whole time reading journals!

The structure of the chapters

In editing this book, we have tried, as far as possible, to draw the chapters together into a single unified text. We were also very mindful that many counsellors and psychotherapists may have limited training in research methods; and that research – like therapy – has its own set of specialist language which is not always clear to non-specialists. Hence, we aimed to achieve certain features and standards across all of our chapters, and asked our authors to take on a particular set of challenges. First, that the writing should be engaging, accessible and stimulating, such that readers would be interested enough to engage with the ideas being presented. Second, that wherever possible the language should be non-technical, jargon-free and direct: accessible to readers who have minimal knowledge of research methodologies or psychology. (Where research terms are used, we have provided a Glossary at the end of the book, and have highlighted the term in bold when first used in a chapter.) Third, that the research should be presented in a non-partisan and open-minded way: one that is able to stand back from any particular orientation or perspective and give a relatively balanced overview of what we know. Fourth, that the text should be written with a spirit of inclusivity and genuine discovery, such that readers from all perspectives will have a faith in the findings that are presented. Fifth, that the text should be based on a comprehensive, in-depth review of research findings in the area under exploration (qualitative as well as quantitative). This might be through a review of primary sources, or through drawing on systematic reviews and meta-analyses where relevant. Sixth, that readers should be given some indication of the certainty of the findings and conclusions presented: Are these things that we can be relatively sure of, is there some uncertainty surrounding it, or is it really only indicative at this stage?

Although there are inevitable differences in the style of each chapter, we have also tried to keep certain things consistent throughout the book. In terms of structure, each chapter begins with approximately four to eight bullet points describing the content of the chapter. This is followed by an introduction which sets out the focus and the significance of the chapter topic. Following the conclusion of the chapter, there is a series of bullet points giving a summary of key findings (except for Chapter 5, where key points are drawn out throughout the chapter). Recommended reading is also given at the end of each chapter, with an annotation for each text explaining why this might be of interest. Every chapter ends with three to six questions for reflection, which invite the reader to consider the key points raised in the chapter. At relevant points in the chapter, there are also sections on implications for practice, which draw out clinical implications of key findings; and chapters also include sections on gaps in research knowledge. These identify areas of counselling and psychotherapy with children and young people where there is insufficient evidence. This not only highlights the ongoing nature of research, but may also be a spur for trainees looking for ideas for their studies.

Difference and diversity across the chapters

As the readers will see, there remain some differences across the chapters and we wanted to allow our authors free reign to write from their particular standpoints.

One particular issue that faces all researchers working in this field is the question of psychiatric diagnosis. Many counsellors and psychotherapists working with children and young people have strong views about the value (or lack of value) of using psychiatric diagnoses, and a number of our chapter authors touch on this issue. However in some fields (such as epidemiology, or treatment outcome studies) almost all of the research to date has been organized in relation to specific psychiatric diagnoses, so that any summary of findings has to follow such a structure. Inevitably there are limitations to this, and in other chapters (such as the chapters on the process of effective therapy) research is not always organized around such diagnostic categories.

There are also some differences in terminology, and although we have tried to standardize methodological terms across the text, we wanted our authors to use the terms they were most comfortable with. Hence, while some of the chapters refer to 'patients', others refer to 'clients'. Equally, some chapters talk of 'treatment' while others use less medical terms such as 'therapy' or 'counselling'.

Throughout the book, we use the term 'child therapy' to cover the wide range of counselling and psychotherapy approaches with children and young people, unless we are describing a study that specifically focuses on one type of counselling or psychotherapy. Likewise, we use the term 'children' to refer to those younger than 11 years, and 'young people' or 'adolescents' to refer to those aged 12–18 years. Where a research paper that is quoted by an author covers ages that are outside these brackets, it will give the age of the study participants. We do not cover research on therapy with parents and infants (under 2 years).

Reflexive statements

Given that, as discussed above, research findings always reflect the biases of their source, we thought it would be useful to finish this introduction by saying something about where we are coming from as editors of the present text.

Nick

I trained as a child psychotherapist at the Anna Freud Centre in London, and was part of the first year-group where the training became part of a professional doctorate at UCL, and so included teaching of research methods and the requirement to carry out a research dissertation. With a background in English literature and the arts, this at first seemed a very alien world to me, and I struggled to get my head around statistics and to see how research and clinical practice could relate in a meaningful way. I was very fortunate to have as my mentors Profs Peter Fonagy and Mary Target, who both embody a commitment to the systematic examination of clinical ideas, not only in regard to treatment outcome, but also in using developmental research to inform the development of clinical practice.

My own doctoral research was supervised by Mary Target, working on a study exploring the long-term follow-up of child analysis, in which I carried out a qualitative analysis of interviews with adults about their memories of being in therapy as children (Midgley and Target, 2005; Midgley, Target, & Smith, 2006). When I started on my research project, I remember that I was struggling as a trainee therapist to work with one particular child in foster care, who kept asking me why he had to come to therapy. At first my tendency was to turn this question back to him, and try to explore why he thought he was coming; but at times this simply enraged him. When I began work on the research project, I was struck by how several of the adults we interviewed about their memories of therapy said that they never really understood why they were taken to therapy as children, or why the sessions happened in the way they did. This was something that had stayed with them for many years, and which they still had strong feelings about. Reflecting on this in my research led me to develop a more open approach in therapy, one in which I always checked out why children thought they were coming to therapy (one recently told me that he had been told he was going to see a dentist!), and I became more confident about sharing my own thoughts and perspectives with the children I work with, and helping them to see – and be curious about – what was going on inside my mind when I said or did certain things. This study also led me to wonder about how other therapists might work with a similar challenge, and before I knew it, I found that systematic curiosity about clinical practice (i.e. research) had become embedded in my very way of being, and has shaped all that I have done in my professional life since.

Jac

As a young person I went to counselling after experiencing a sudden and life-threatening neurological illness, and being quite shell-shocked about re-entering the world of 15 year olds at school doing their GCSEs. This first experience of therapy had helpful elements but also reinforced some of my heightened state of confusion –

looking back I realize there was a lot that was unsaid between me and the therapist, who I experienced as quite cold and detached – I left feeling I may have wasted her time and she probably had kids with 'real' problems to deal with. As an adult I worked in the psychiatric system and then trained in person-centred therapy, and later cognitive behavioural therapy. Although my interest in various therapies remains, my congruence as a therapist lies with person-centred values. As a researcher, learning about the history of psychology, the philosophy of science, and then being involved in hearing voices (sometimes known as verbal hallucination) research, has taught me to be wary of taking any findings out of context, and to never be quick to label. This education has also told me that the medical model of psychological problems is just one hypothesis among many, and I prefer to define problems, including those that children and young people face, as 'problems of living' and talk about them in their more everyday sense – 'bullying', 'divorce', 'relationship with father', 'feeling sad'. In terms of research methods, I do have favourites and these usually include those that capture therapeutic processes in real-time, such as conversation analysis.

Mick

I trained initially in person-centred therapy, and then went on to study as an existential psychotherapist. So my practice and writing has always had a strongly relational emphasis, and I've been more wary of highly technical practices. I have also tended to be fairly ambivalent towards psychodynamic therapies. In part, this probably comes from my own experiences as a young person in psychoanalytic psychotherapy at the Tavistock Institute, where I felt that the analytical focus on the here-and-now relationship overshadowed my desire to get some direct help and practical support. I also tend to prefer approaches that emphasize a mutual, dialogical relationship, as opposed to those in which the therapist is the 'knower' and the client 'the known'. Having said that, as Nick indicates, I am aware of the many moves within the psychodynamic field towards more relational practices, and ones that place increasing emphasis on shared decision-making with children and young people. I find these developments very exciting, and strive to be open to a wide plurality of therapeutic approaches (see Cooper & McLeod, 2011; Cooper & Dryden, 2016). In terms of research methods, I am also fairly pluralistic in my views. However, through writing and researching the original *Essential research findings* book, I did find myself increasingly drawn towards research with clear pragmatic implications. That is, research that simply said things about what helped or did not help clients, even if it was coming from a positivist, mechanistic standpoint.

Conclusion

Talia has begun to talk. Awkwardly and uncomfortably, but she has said a bit more about losing her nan, how it really upset her, and how she finds it difficult to talk to people about what she feels. She doesn't like people, she says. They're always interfering – never really listening to her. Her mum is the best example of that, says Talia, criticizing and complaining. But she goes on to say that maybe, perhaps a bit, she can understand why her mum's always been so angry. Her dad was violent, and when he finally left, Talia knows her mum had so much on and 'not much of a life'.

A few days later in supervision, Talia's therapist reflects on how to help her take the work forward. It feels like supporting and encouraging Talia to talk about her family members is helpful. It seems like the warmth of the therapist is supporting her to open up. The therapist also talks through some other ideas that might be useful for Talia: problem-solving, supporting her to take the lead in therapy, and making sense of Talia's way of relating in terms of her attachment style. Here, as the therapist talks through these possibilities, research and practice, evidence and experience, mix and merge.

Ultimately, the aim of this book is to contribute to the pool of resources that inform your practice: to help you to be able to draw on research findings, as well the many other invaluable understandings, ideas and experiences that you may have. As with Talia, given the complexities and the challenges of the children and young people we may work with, the more knowledge we have, the more we may be able to help.

Recommended reading

Cooper, M. (2008). *Essential research findings in counselling and psychotherapy: The facts are friendly*. London: Sage. Comprehensive review of research findings in the adult therapy field, identifying key domains of research evidence.

Fonagy, P., Cottrell, D., Phillips, J., Bevington, D., Glasser, D., & Allison, E. (2015). *What works for whom? A critical review of treatments for children and adolescence* (2nd ed.). New York: Guilford Press. Definitive review of evidence-based therapies for different psychological problems in childhood.

McLeod, J. (2013). *Doing research in counselling and psychotherapy* (3rd ed.). London: Sage. Concise introduction to research methods and issues in the field.

Questions for reflection

- What would you consider the value, and limitations, of research findings in your own work with children and young people?
- What biases and assumptions about what works for children and young people do you bring to reading this book?
- What kind of research questions would come out of your own experience of working as a counsellor or therapist with children and young people?

References

Boisvert, C. M., & Faust, D. (2006). Practicing psychologists' knowledge of general psychotherapy research findings: Implications for science–practice relations. *Professional Psychology: Research and Practice*, 37(6), 708–716.

Cochrane, A. (1972). *Effectiveness and efficiency: Random reflections on health services*. London: Nuffield Provincial Hospitals Trust.

Cooper, M. (2008). *Essential research findings in counselling and psychotherapy.* London: Sage.

Cooper, M., & Dryden, W. (Eds.). (2016). *Handbook of pluralistic counselling and psychotherapy.* London: Sage.

Cooper, M., & McLeod, J. (2011). *Pluralistic counselling and psychotherapy.* London: Sage.

Darlington, Y., & Scott, D. (2002). *Qualitative research in practice: Stories from the field.* Buckingham: Open University Press.

Midgley, N., & Target, M. (2005). Recollections of being in child psychoanalysis: A qualitative study of a long-term follow-up project. *Psychoanalytic Study of the Child, 60,* 157–177.

Midgley, N., Target, M., & Smith, J. A. (2006). The outcome of child psychoanalysis from the patient's point of view: A qualitative analysis of a long-term follow-up study. *Psychology and Psychotherapy: Theory, Practice, Research, 79,* 257–269.

Morrow-Bradley, C., & Elliott, R. (1986). Utilization of psychotherapy research by practicing psychotherapists. *American Psychologist, 41,* 188–197.

Oakley, A., Gough, D., Oliver, S., & Thomas, J. (2005). The politics of evidence and methodology: Lessons from the EPPI-Centre. *Evidence and Policy, 1*(1), 5–31.

Sackett, D., Rosenberg, W., Muir Gray, J., Haynes, R., & Richardson, W. (1996). Editorial: Evidence-based medicine: what it is and what it isn't. *British Medical Journal, 312,* 71–7.

2

EPIDEMIOLOGY: ARE MENTAL HEALTH PROBLEMS IN CHILDREN AND YOUNG PEOPLE REALLY A BIG ISSUE?

ANN HAGELL AND BARBARA MAUGHAN

This chapter discusses

- What we mean by mental health problems in childhood
- How common mental health problems are in childhood and adolescence
- Ways of measuring child and adolescent mental health problems
- How mental health problems in childhood and adolescence develop
- Why mental health problems in children and young people are important
- What kinds of services are available to help

Introduction

Mental health problems in children and adolescents are common and distressing. Although the majority of children and young people rate their wellbeing as good most of the time, a significant minority will suffer from some kind of mental health problem as they grow up. Prevention, early intervention and treatment are all important for improving children's outcomes.

Mental health problems in childhood encompass a broad range of disorders that affect thinking, feeling or mood, and have an impact on everyday functioning. Those most frequent problems in the childhood years include anxiety and depression, eating disorders, conduct disorder (serious antisocial behaviour), substance use disorders, attention deficit and hyperactivity disorder (ADHD), and difficulties associated with autism spectrum disorder. During childhood and adolescence there can also be the early signs of the precursors of rarer problems such as personality disorders or bipolar disorders.

In this chapter we will focus on specific mental health problems, rather than more generic emotional difficulties such as responses to life events like bereavement. All children will experience the latter to some degree in their lives, and these kinds of problems are too diffuse to be captured in epidemiological research except perhaps though measurements of wellbeing and happiness, which we do not cover here.

It has been estimated that three-quarters of young adults with mental health disorders will first have met criteria for disorder before the age of 18 (Kim-Cohen, Caspi, Moffitt, Harrington, Milne, & Poutton, 2003). Mental health problems have important implications for every aspect of young people's lives, including their ability to engage with education, make and keep friends, engage in constructive family relationships and find their own way in the world. Yet there is stigma associated with discussing the issues, families often feel isolated, and getting help can be a challenge as services are limited. We need to understand the pattern of child and adolescent mental health disorders in order to target interventions and, where possible, help prevent problems from arising.

How common are mental health problems in childhood and adolescence?

How do we know the answer to this question?

The methods of epidemiology offer a way of describing and measuring child and adolescent mental health problems. **Epidemiology** is the study of the distribution and determinants of health and disease in populations. The key measures of interest to us here are incidence and prevalence. **Incidence** relates to new occurrences; how many children develop mental health problems? This might be measured across childhood, or over a set period of time such as across the course of one year. **Prevalence** relates to existing occurrences; what proportion of children have a mental health problem at any given point ('point prevalence')?

The measures used for assessing mental health problems and the methods used for surveying populations are critical to our confidence in the findings of epidemiological studies, and affect our ability to generalize from the findings. The standard systems for measuring child and adolescent mental health problems are the diagnostic systems of the American Psychiatric Association (Diagnostic and Statistical Manual [DSM] of Mental Disorders, 2013), and of the World Health Organization (International Classification of Diseases [ICD]). The advantage of these classification systems is that they are widely accepted, used in much research, and provide a 'common language' for the field. However, they can give the impression of a fixed set of criteria, when in fact they are revised and changed as research evolves. Much of what upsets and challenges children and young people is also hard to fit within standard classification systems (a point we return to later), and reliance on the diagnostic criteria can direct research and treatment to focus just on the more classifiable problems.

However, it is important to recognize how important these systems are for how we think about young people's mental health disorders, and there are a number of different ways of assessing whether children meet the criteria for a disorder in the

DSM or ICD systems. The best use direct semi-structured interviews with children and/or their parents. However, other data are available from surveys that draw on questionnaires rather than interviews, and that use other ways of rating mental health problems other than the DSM and ICD systems. As we do not know as much as we would like about the incidence and prevalence of child and adolescent mental health problems, we have to rely in part on this wider body of research too.

We can also use data from **longitudinal studies**, following up groups of children over a period of several years, to map how disease unfolds and the factors involved in the course that the problems take.

Box 2.1   Key studies: The Avon Longitudinal Study of Parents and Children (ALSPAC)

ALSPAC, also known as the *Children of the 90s* study, has followed approximately 14,000 children in the Bristol area of England since the early 1990s, linking successive waves of data collection to build a picture of the influences on their outcomes as they grow into adulthood. It has resulted in over 1,000 academic papers and a number of important findings, many relating to mental health. Over the years, the children and their families have completed numerous questionnaires, given biological samples for genetic analysis, and allowed their medical and educational records to be followed. A new study, COCO90s, is now beginning to follow the children of the *Children of the 90s*.

Findings from the study include, for example, important data on the associations between mothers' binge drinking and behaviour problems in early childhood; the early warning signs in children and adolescents of increased risk of schizophrenia; and the links between self-harm at 16 and a range of health and attainment outcomes at 16–21. These kinds of findings help to focus efforts to identify issues early and intervene to prevent problems from getting worse.

See www.bristol.ac.uk/alspac/ for more details.

There are two key issues about measurement – is it accurate, and does it reflect what we see in practice? Turning first to accuracy, we might for example have questions about the accuracy of parents' reports on their children, which is often how younger children are assessed. Or we might wonder, if we ask young people today about their problems, are the answers comparable to those of young people 20 years ago? What difference does it make to surveys if attitudes to mental health problems change over time and people feel more able to admit difficulties? There is now a large literature addressing many of these issues of accuracy, and we return to the question of time trends below. We know quite a lot, for example, about when parental reporting is and is not accurate. Parents may be better informants for problems that are easier to observe, such as attention and hyperactivity, rather than for internalizing difficulties such as depression (De Los Reyes et al., 2015; Grills & Ollendick, 2002; Van der Ende, Verhulst, & Tiemeier, 2012).

The difficulty is that accuracy comes with the amount of time that can be spent in assessment, and often front-line practice is pressurized for time. In addition, accuracy comes with training, and the real challenge has been to develop ways of assessing child mental health problems that do not require qualifications in child mental health, so they can be used, for example, in youth work settings. There have been interesting developments lately in improving community-based screening for difficulties. For example, Mental Health First Aid (MHFA) training alerts non-specialists to crucial warning signs of mental ill health that require professional assessment, although this is perhaps more relevant to understanding how to manage risk rather than how to measure frequency of problems. Developed in Australia in 2000, MHFA has now been delivered to over 100,000 professionals in the UK, including teachers.

Box 2.2 Common ways of measuring child and adolescent mental health problems

Diagnostic interviews

Different styles of interview have been developed to assess common mental health problems (Angold, Erkanli, Copeland, Goodman, Fisher, & Costello, 2012):

- Structured: for example, the Diagnostic Interview Schedule for Children (DISC-IV)
- Interviewer-based/semi-structured: for example, the Child and Adolescent Psychiatric Assessment (CAPA)
- Structured + expert judgement: for example, the Development and Well-Being Assessment (DAWBA)

These interviews typically take between half an hour and an hour to complete.

There are versions for pre-schoolers, school-age children and adolescents, and young adults. Information can be collected from parents/carers, teachers and young people themselves; these interviews can also be used in clinical settings.

Information is collected about the frequency, duration and severity of symptoms, and associated impairments. Computer algorithms (confirmed by review by experts in the DAWBA) are then used to generate DSM/ICD diagnoses and symptom counts.

More specialized interviews have been developed to assess less common disorders (for example, the Autism Diagnostic Interview [ADI] for autistic spectrum disorders).

Questionnaires

Standardized, reliable questionnaires have also been developed to assess many specific aspects of child mental health.

There are also well-established 'broad band' measures that assess the range of common difficulties, and are often used as screening instruments. The most widely used (available in a range of languages) are:

- The Strengths and Difficulties Questionnaire (SDQ) www.sdqinfo.com/. The SDQ includes 25 main questions assessing conduct and emotional problems, hyperactivity, peer difficulties and prosocial behaviours; it also includes a brief impact supplement. Versions are available to assess pre-schoolers and school-age children, and for completion by parents, teachers and young people aged 11 and older.

(Continued)

(Continued)

- The Child Behavior Checklist (CBCL) www.aseba.org/. The CBCL includes just over 100 questions, and assesses a range of syndromes (anxious/depressed, withdrawn/depressed, rule-breaking behaviour, aggressive behaviour, attention problems, thought problems, somatic complaints, social problems); it also includes DSM-oriented scales. It is part of a suite of instruments for children of different ages, and for completion by parents, teachers and young people.
- The Revised Children's Anxiety and Depression Scale (RCADS), assesses a range of different subtypes of anxiety and depression, providing two total scores and various subscale scores. Several versions exist, including one with 47 items and one with 25. Again there are separate versions for completion by children and adolescents and their parents (Chorpita, Yim, Moffitt, Umemoto, & Francis, 2000).

The second issue, that of whether the diagnostic categories reflect what we see in practice, is perhaps more difficult to answer, as we lack good representative data on the types of cases that do not meet the criteria for formal psychiatric service input. These may involve children and young people who are seen in general practice, or in voluntary sector organizations working with young people in difficulty. In these cases, counsellors and other practitioners often reflect that children and young people might still have severe problems even if they do not fall neatly into a formal diagnosis. Epidemiological studies reporting on formal diagnoses may not represent the full range of complicated issues young people can present with. Overlaps of disorders are also very common. One nationally representative study of over 10,000 American adolescents concluded that approximately 40 per cent of those with one class of formal disorder (anxiety, behaviour problems, mood problems, substance misuse) also met the criteria for a second disorder (Merikangas et al., 2010).

However, the measurement systems we have, leading to representative epidemiological data, are the best available and do give useful estimates of the proportions of the child and adolescent population who are likely to need some kind of support and help as they make the transition through childhood and adolescence and into adulthood. Using these standard systems helps us to compare across different studies, age groups or geographical areas, and some of the more user-friendly screening questionnaires, such as the Strengths and Difficulties Questionnaire (Goodman, 1999), are now widely used across all sectors dealing with children and young people.

Box 2.3   How do we know the difference between mental health problems and the ordinary ups and downs of adolescence?

Moodiness and irritability are of course classic symptoms of adolescence. We know from recent neuropsychological studies that there are many ways in which adolescents' brains are still developing which influence their perspective on the world and affect their behaviour.

It is difficult for young people, parents, teachers and others to know when ordinary teenage ups and downs become a mental health problem that needs intervention.

There are no easy answers to the question, but there are some things to look out for that would suggest a problem is more than just transient moodiness:

- The problem is persistent – ongoing sadness, anxiety or irritability
- There is a sense of hopelessness and not being able to enjoy regular activities, with possibly recurrent thoughts of death and suicide (not necessarily with any action plan)
- The young person regularly expresses negative, distressing or unusual thoughts
- Physical symptoms are also present – difficulties with sleeping (too much, or insomnia), changes to appetite, heart palpitations
- Mood interferes with the ability to do regular daily things
- There are changes in performance at school, college or work

If young people show several of these difficulties on most days, for two weeks or longer, it is likely that more support is needed and possibly intervention.

Useful information on these issues for parents and children can be found in a number of online resources, including:

- MindEd, a free educational resource on children and young people's mental health for all adults, including a range of e-learning modules, www.minded.org.uk/
- The Site, an online guide to life for 16–25 year olds, including useful pages on mental health problems, www.thesite.org/
- Young Minds, a national charity promoting children and young people's mental health, with extensive resources and a parents helpline, www.youngminds.org.uk/

What do we know from surveys?

The overwhelming and consistent thing that we know from surveys is that child and adolescent mental health problems are common, and always have been – at least, for as long as we have been asking the question. Table 2.1 presents evidence from the last UK representative survey of rates of different mental health disorders in the general population of children and young people (Green, McGinnity, Meltzer, Ford, & Goodman, 2005). The survey was undertaken for the Office for National Statistics (ONS) in 2004. The data suggest that the most common mental health problems from age 5 to 16 are conduct disorders (antisocial behaviour), and emotional disorders (including depression and anxiety). Hyperkinetic disorders (including ADHD) are the third most common group of problems, indicated by poor attention, hyperactivity and impulsivity across a number of settings, home and school. Overall, emotional disorders are more common in girls across this age range, and conduct disorders are more common in boys. At any one time, we can expect nearly 10 per cent of children between 5 and 16 years to have a measurable mental health problem.

The reported prevalence of mental health problems in the 2004 ONS survey varied by ethnicity. Rates of mental health problems were higher in some ethnic minority groups (Black), and lower in others (Indian, Pakistani and Bangladeshi). This is a complicated question, because as well as reflecting real differences in rates of problems, the findings may also reflect cultural differences in measurement and assessment; but this is a fairly generally reported pattern and thus an important issue to

Table 2.1 Prevalence of mental disorders by age and sex, Great Britain, 2004.[a]

Type of disorder	5–10 year olds (%)			11–16 year olds (%)			All children (%)		
	Boys	**Girls**	**All**	**Boys**	**Girls**	**All**	**Boys**	**Girls**	**All**
Emotional disorders	2.2	2.5	2.4	4.0	6.1	5.0	3.1	4.3	3.7
Conduct disorders	6.9	2.8	4.9	8.1	5.1	6.6	7.5	3.9	5.8
Hyperkinetic disorders	2.7	0.4	1.6	2.4	0.4	1.4	2.6	0.4	1.5
Less common disorders	2.2	0.4	1.3	1.6	1.1	1.4	1.9	0.8	1.3
Any disorder	10.2	5.1	7.7	12.6	10.3	11.5	11.4	7.8	9.6
Base (weighted)[b]	*2,010*	*1,916*	*3,926*	*2,101*	*1,950*	*4,051*	*4,111*	*3,866*	*7,977*

[a] Prevalence rates are based on the ICD-10 Classification of Mental and Behavioural Disorders with strict impairment criteria – the disorder causing distress to the child or having a considerable impact on the child's day-to-day life.

[b] The weighted base represents statistical adjustments made so that the sample represents the total population.

Source: Green et al. (2005).

keep in sight. The distribution of disorders also appeared to be associated with social background. Young people living in households with higher levels of parental educational qualifications had lower levels of mental disorders.

Hyperkinetic disorders include attention deficit and hyperactivity disorder, and the key symptoms are inattention, impulsiveness and hyperactivity. This group of disorders is less common than emotional or conduct disorders, affecting between 0.4 and 2.7 per cent of children depending on age and gender. Rates are consistently higher in boys than girls.

Two other important groups of disorders include eating disorders and autism spectrum disorders. Eating disorders often start in adolescence, and it is estimated that around one in 250 females and one in 2,000 males will experience anorexia nervosa, usually as an adolescent or young adult, and that around five times this number will suffer from bulimia nervosa (National Collaborating Centre for Mental Health, 2012). Anorexia is in fact the most fatal mental health disorder, with an estimated mortality rate of around 10 per cent (Arcelus, Mitchell, Wales, & Nielsen, 2011). However, good representative community surveys are rare.

Turning to autism, the new DSM-5, published in 2013, has drawn together the various diagnoses of autism, autism spectrum and Asperger's into an umbrella category of 'autistic spectrum disorder'. The Green et al. (2005) study suggested a prevalence rate of around 1 per cent for these kinds of communication difficulties. Autism is perhaps better characterized as a neurodevelopmental condition rather than a psychiatric disorder, and consists of abnormal social communication and patterns of behaviour. There are ongoing debates as to whether it is best represented as a spectrum or a set of distinct conditions with similar symptoms, and there are also debates over the point at which communication difficulties should be classified as a disorder. There is no definitive test for autism, and growing awareness of the condition and changing diagnostic criteria make it difficult to estimate prevalence or determine whether there are rises or not. However, it is useful to note that up to 70 per cent of 10–14 year old children with autism have been shown to have co-occurring psychiatric disorders such as social anxiety disorder and attention deficit hyperactivity disorder (Simonoff, Pickles, Charman, Chandler, Loucas, & Baird, 2008).

Box 2.4 Comorbity: A key debate

Children and young people will often show symptoms of more than one disorder at the same time. As we have already noted, comorbidity, as this is known, is very common, which may indicate that there are issues with how the classification systems are separating out disorders that actually occur together, or perhaps suggesting that there are more general underlying vulnerabilities that could increase risk for multiple disorders. Indeed, some researchers have queried the assumption that mental disorders can be viewed as distinct, categorical conditions; Caspi et al. (2013) used longitudinal data from the Dunedin study to demonstrate that one 'General Psychopathology' dimension (the 'p' factor) may be a more useful way to view the structure of psychiatric disorders.

Other sources of information

As well as national representative surveys, there are other useful sources of information about children and young people's mental health difficulties. We can illustrate some of these by taking the example of self-harm. Self-harm (deliberate cutting or scratching) is often a symptom of depression or anxiety, and causes intense concern for families and schools. However, it is a very private behaviour and a very sensitive topic, and thus difficult to subject to surveys. Estimates of the rates of self-harm in adolescent girls are available from several large-scale surveys such as the English version of the Health Behaviour in School Aged Children Survey (HBSC), the Avon Longitudinal Study (ALSPAC) and various more localized school-based surveys. These suggest rates from around 14 per cent of pupils aged 15–16 (O'Connor, Rasmussen, Miles, & Hawton, 2009) up to 22 per cent (Brooks, Magnusson, Klemera, Chester, Spencer, & Smeeton, 2015). Rates are up to three times higher in young women than young men (Brooks et al., 2015).

A minority of young people who self-harm end up in hospital; estimates suggest that hospital admissions represent around one in eight cases in the community (Hawton, Saunders, & O'Connor, 2012). However the routine collection of hospital admission statistics ('Hospital Episode Statistics') does allow us to look at trends over time, even though they may represent the tip of an iceberg. In 2014 there were 41,921 hospitalizations for self-harm (self-poisoning and other methods) among 10–24 year olds in England. Rates of hospital admissions for all kinds of self-harm per 100,000 population aged 10–24 have risen from 330 in 2007/8 to 367 in 2013/14 (Hagell, Coleman, & Brooks, 2015). These different data sources demonstrate some of the difficulties of trying to piece together the full picture, particularly for such a private and stigmatized topic as self-harm, much of which receives no treatment. The data also show the importance of using lots of different indicators from different parts of the system when trying to work out prevalence and whether problems are increasing or not.

Trends over time and international comparisons

There is much debate about whether today's generation of young people is more anxious, depressed and stressed than previous generations (Collishaw, Maughan, Goodman, & Pickles, 2004; Hagell, 2012). The evidence suggests that there was a rise in emotional and behavioural problems over the last three or so decades of the twentieth century up to 2000 (Collishaw et al., 2004) but epidemiological data in the early 2000s suggested a levelling out (Maughan, Collishaw, Meltzer, & Goodman, 2008). In fact, in the UK, there has not been a good, national representative survey of child and adolescent mental health problems since 2004, although a new government-funded survey is currently planned. This will reveal what has happened in the intervening decade or so, and whether the anecdotal accounts of rises reported by front-line staff in schools, the health service and the voluntary sector have been reflected in the population data.

Even if good data are available, interpreting time trends is very difficult. If increases in problems are seen, we might suggest that we just diagnose more, or that our criteria for diagnosis have got wider, or that perceptions of 'normal' have changed. However there are methodological checks and balances that can be brought to bear to make us more confident that what we see in the data is indeed what has happened. Thus, for example, in the Collishaw et al. study (see Box 2.5), the strengths of associations between psychiatric symptoms and poor outcomes later in adulthood remained similar over time for three different birth cohorts from 1974 to 1999, suggesting that the results were not attributable to changes in the thresholds of what is counted as a problem. It seemed the increasing time trends were not, for example, the result of an increasing tendency for parents to rate teenagers as having problems, but were instead the result of changes in frequency of problems. The other check is to make sure that different sources of data reflect similar patterns; we saw this with the data on self-harm.

Box 2.5   Key studies: Time trends in adolescent mental health

Collishaw et al. (2004) analysed data from three national surveys of the UK general population, drawing on data from three huge studies of population samples. The focus of the study was 15–16 year olds in **1974** (from the National Child Development Study), in **1986** (from the 1970 Birth Cohort Study) and in **1999** (from the British Child and Adolescent Mental Health Survey).

In each survey, parents completed comparable questionnaires about their children's mental health symptoms. The results showed:

- Adolescent conduct problems showed a continuous rise for both boys and girls over the whole 25-year period.
- Reports of emotional problems (such as depression and anxiety) increased for both girls and boys from the mid-1980s to 1999.
- There were few systematic trends in adolescent hyperactivity over the 25-year period for either boys or girls, with no clear indication that levels are either increasing or decreasing.

In an interesting example of more recent time trends in behaviour problems, the international Health Behaviour in School Aged Children Survey (HBSC) has collected data on fighting from over 30 countries over a number of years. Looking at the 2002–10 data, Pickett et al. (2013) concluded that there were declines over time in two-thirds of the countries involved, including the UK and USA. Rises were seen particularly in countries that had suffered severe economic crises during the inter-vening years, such as Greece and Spain.

How do mental health problems in childhood and adolescence develop?

Patterns of mental health problems across the lifespan

It is now widely recognized that mental health problems have roots very early in development. Epidemiological studies also suggest that different groups of disorders start at different ages in childhood and adolescence. The neurodevelopmental disorders (including autism spectrum disorders) show the earliest ages at onset, but surveys of adults as well as children find that up to half of all specific phobias, along with separation anxiety disorders and ADHD, will typically have emerged by age 7. Many oppositional and conduct problems also become evident in the late pre-school and early school years.

Surveys of mental health problems in pre-schoolers are a relatively recent development; where they have been undertaken, however, they show that the structure of mental health problems in 3 and 4 year olds is quite similar to that in young school-age children, and that rates of disorder are quite similar too (Angold & Egger, 2007).

As young people approach adolescence – and especially perhaps the onset of puberty – a new set of mental health problems begins to emerge. Depression, social anxieties and eating disorders are among the most important of these. Clinically significant depressive disorders are, of course, found in some younger children, but rates are generally low, and boys are as likely to be affected as girls. From around age 13, however, rates begin to rise quite markedly, and the female preponderance typical of adult depression begins to emerge. By adulthood, women are approxi-mately twice as likely to have depression (Bebbington, 1996). Eating disorders tend to start in the mid-teens and routine Hospital Episode Statistics in the UK show that young people aged 10–19 account for more than half of hospital admissions (Health and Social Care Information Centre, 2014). The largest number of hospital admissions with a primary diagnosis of eating disorders is at age 15 (Hagell et al., 2015). Rates of conduct problems and delinquency also rise from the early to mid-teens, and most disorders associated with alcohol and drug abuse typically start later in adolescence. The early states of psychotic disorders begin to emerge in the late teens, as does panic disorder – which for reasons that are still not well understood, appears to be rare if not non-existent in childhood.

What do we know about the contributing factors?

A vast volume of research has explored risk factors for child mental health problems, and an equally wide range of potential contributory factors have been identified.

We should note at the outset that most of this evidence is correlational in nature. **Correlational studies** infer a relationship between two variables based on the fact they occur together, but usually we cannot assume that one caused the other. For example, if playing violent computer games is associated with increased antisocial behaviour in a **cross-sectional study**, it is impossible to tell which comes first; indeed, both might be caused by a third, unmeasured factor. The experimental studies that would be needed to identify **causal relationships** are rarely feasible in psychiatric research (or indeed in studies of other aspects of human behaviour), though many approaches have been developed to help strengthen **causal inference**, such as taking advantage of natural experiments where, perhaps, one class of schoolchildren is exposed to some kind of intervention when another is not.

The first general message to emerge from research on the causes of mental health problems is that they are multifactorial in origin: a wide range of influences, spanning individual child characteristics, family and peer group influences, and wider social and cultural factors, are all likely to be implicated. Ecological theories of development (see, for example, Bronfenbrenner, 1979) highlight the interplay among different levels of risk, some very near to, some more distant from, the child (see Figure 2.1).

Risks may vary at different stages in development, and for different children with apparently similar problems; indeed, there seems to be marked variability in response to almost all known risks, suggesting that many children also benefit from protective or resilience-related factors that help offset the adverse effects of exposure to risks (for example, Rutter, 2012). A second broad conclusion is that individual risk factors rarely operate in isolation: most disorders probably result from a complex interplay between different types of risk, including biological as well as psychological and social influences (for example, Rutter, Moffitt, & Caspi, 2006). And finally, though some risk factors are relatively specific to particular disorders, many show associations with a broad spectrum of child outcomes. Child abuse and neglect is an example here.

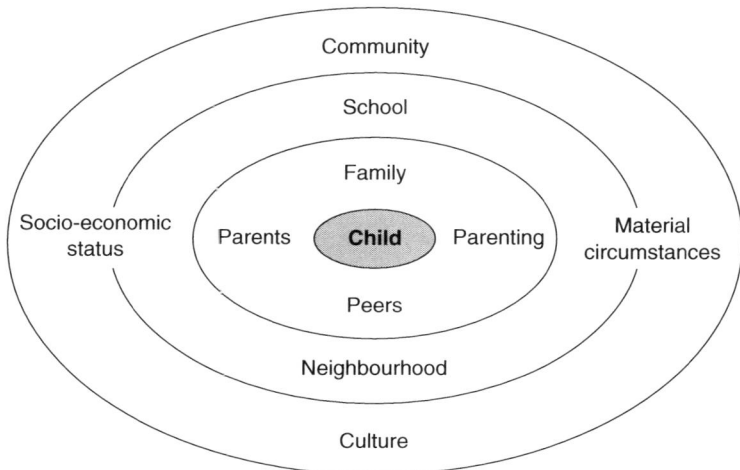

Figure 2.1 Factors influencing mental health problems

Box 2.6   Risk factors for child mental health problems

- **Individual child characteristics**: temperament; neurobiological factors (including stress regulation mechanisms); neuropsychological and neurophysiological factors (including brain structure and functioning); information processing and social cognition.
- **Family-level factors**: heritable influence (including gene–environment interplay); prenatal and perinatal influences; parenting; attachment; family structure and functioning; family poverty and disadvantage; abuse and neglect.
- **Influences beyond the family**: peers; schooling and education; neighbourhood; wider social influences; life events. These may have direct impacts on parents and children, or moderate other patterns of influence so that, for example, parenting is more challenging in some social contexts than others.

Genetic influences

- Many mental health problems run in families; genetic factors contribute to these effects.
- Although biological markers have not always been established, some disorders (such as ADHD) appear to be highly heritable, while others (such as many anxiety disorders) show less strong genetic effects.
- New genetic influences come on stream across development.
- Most heritable influences on mental health problems seem likely to stem from multiple genes, each of small effect.
- Gene–environment interplay is important: genetic factors may affect susceptibility to environmental risks, or influence risk exposure.
- Epigenetic mechanisms (such as DNA methylation) are responsive to environmental influences.

See Thapar, Pine, Leckman, Scott, Snowling and Taylor (2015) *Rutter's child and adolescent psychiatry* (6th ed.) for more information on risk factors and genetic influences.

Box 2.7   Gaps in research: Why is adolescence such a risky period for the onset of anxiety and mood disorders?

There are a number of hypotheses about why anxiety, panic and depression start to emerge in the teens, but we are not absolutely certain. This is partly because experimental studies are extremely hard to do with such sensitive topics. We have to make assumptions from cross-sectional data that cannot tell us about causality, or try to unpick the picture from longitudinal studies which might have been designed to address rather different research questions; but the suggestions include:

- The teenage years see an increase in stress as young people face educational pressures.
- The transition to being an autonomous adult is also potentially stressful.
- Peer pressures can ratchet up the anxiety levels, particularly perhaps for young women.
- Adolescent brains are still undergoing development and perhaps some aspect of the structural changes makes the teen brain particularly susceptible to mood changes.

Why is it important to have good information about mental health problems in young people?

As we have seen, mental health problems in children and young people are common. Undoubtedly they cause distress, both for the individual and also their family. In some cases, such as depression and anorexia, they may lead to death. In fact over half of deaths for those aged 15–19 are attributable to external causes including suicide and violent deaths, transport injuries, drowning and fire, and many of those who die from suicide have not had contact with mental health services (Wolfe, Macfarlane, Donkin, Marmot, & Viner, 2014). There is considerable continuity between childhood and adult problems (Jones, 2013). As we stated at the outset, it has been estimated that half of all lifetime cases of psychiatric disorders start by age 14, and three-quarters by age 24 (Kessler, Bergulund, Demler, Jin, Merikangas, & Walters, 2005), and some estimates suggest the majority start before age 18 (Kim-Cohen et al., 2003). As a result of both their commonness and their links to adult health, mental health problems are a major contributor to the global burden of disease (Whiteford et al., 2013) and untreated problems are likely to be very expensive for health services both at the time of diagnosis, but also as young people grow into adulthood. Drawing on British national survey data, Snell et al. (2013) estimated that the additional health, social care and education costs associated with child psychiatric disorders totalled £1.47 billion in 2008, mostly relating to costs borne by the education sector.

Untreated mental health problems obviously also have a large cost for the individual. In a recent analysis of the economic impacts of youth mental health, Knapp et al. (2016) analysed data from the 2000 Adult Psychiatric Morbidity Survey and found that young people aged 16–25 with mental health issues were significantly more likely to be not in employment, education and training than their peers, and to be almost twice as likely to be on welfare benefits.

Yet mental health problems, as is set out more fully in Chapters 4 and 5, are treatable. The National Institute for Health and Clinical Excellence (NICE) provides a range of pathways and advice for tackling mental health in children and young people, including detailed information on treating depression in people under 18 (National Institute for Health and Clinical Excellence, 2005).

Mental health services for children and young people

Improving mental health outcomes is clearly on the international agenda. In 2013, the World Health Organization launched its Mental Health Action Plan 2013–20, with targets including a 20 per cent increase in service coverage for mental health problems, and a reduction of 10 per cent to suicide rates (WHO, 2013). The mental health of young people is subject to considerable policy discussion in the UK at the time of writing, partly as a result of the House of Commons Health Committee report on the topic in October 2014, and the government report *Future in mind*, published in 2015 following the work of the Children and Young People's Mental Health Taskforce (Department of Heath, 2015). There is a consensus that services are not always available when and where they are needed. There is considerable emphasis on the importance of all kinds of service providers in this, not simply statutory CAMHS but also including social care, the voluntary sector, schools, colleges and universities.

What's available?

Other chapters in this book deal more fully with treatment options for child and adolescent mental health problems, but in the context of this chapter it is useful to provide a brief outline of what is available and some of the issues as they currently stand. In the UK, child and adolescent mental health is dealt with by a wide range of different professionals in different settings. Traditionally these have been ordered into 'Tiers' to help us conceptualize them:

Tier 1: universal services provided by non-specialists such as primary care workers and school nurses

Tier 2: specialized mental health workers offering support in the community, including, for example, working in GPs' surgeries and voluntary sector providers

Tier 3: specialist mental health professionals working in multidisciplinary teams based in a local clinic: what is often referred to as CAMHS (child and adolescent mental health services) although CAMHS is wider than just Tier 3

Tier 4: specialized day and inpatient units.

Wolpert et al. (2015) have suggested a new way to conceptualize this range of services which focuses more on the kinds of inputs that individuals will need. Their 'Thrive' model identifies five needs-based groupings – the 'thriving' majority who need no external help and have no, or very minimal, mental health difficulties; a group who can, or choose to, manage their difficulties with minimal external support; people who are getting goal-focused help and intervention; people getting more extensive treatment including inpatient services; and people who need risk management and crisis response but who, for a multitude of reasons, could not make use of active change interventions.

NICE provides the overarching guidance on how to treat mental health problems, and has distinct treatment pathways for those under 18 for treatment of depression and anxiety, for example. These guide the interventions on offer, and essentially suggest 'talking' treatments should always be the first line of intervention with this age group, with recourse to medication only alongside a talking treatment or if other options have failed. For example, statutory CAMHS will usually offer a range of interventions including a course of cognitive behavioural therapy, art therapy, child psychotherapy or family therapy, as well as medication.

The 'treatment gap'

At the time of writing there are no national datasets in the UK that tell us how many children and young people are seen for mental health problems in different parts of the health system, and there is also a lack of data on services provided by others including, for example, school counsellors and voluntary sector services in the community. The majority of children with difficulties will initially be seen in primary care. General practitioners (GPs) are often the first port of call for families facing difficulties with their young children and teenagers. Training in child and adolescent mental health is not part of the compulsory GP training programme and so the expertise of the family doctor will vary.

The options for GPs for onward referral are also fairly limited. The statutory CAMHS have limited capacity and high thresholds; it is often the case that only children in crisis will meet the criteria for assessment and treatment. The NHS estimates that 1,400 per 100,000 of the population aged 0–19 will be referred to CAMHS (NHS Benchmarking Network, 2013). Specialized inpatient beds are extremely limited, with approximately 1,400 across the whole of England.

As we have suggested that at least 10 per cent of the adolescent population (and around 5 per cent of the younger child population) will have mental health symptoms that are of a level that warrants treatment, there is clearly a fairly substantial 'treatment gap'. It has been estimated from a large national survey that over half of 12–15 year olds with mental health issues have no contact with services for these problems, and that this gap is wider for adolescents and young adults than any other age group (Knapp et al., 2016). In a survey of 3,750 young people aged 12–16 in UK secondary schools, only 5 per cent of those at high risk of depression or self-harm had seen specialist CAMHS in the previous six months. Among those with probable depression, 79 per cent had seen their GP and 5 per cent had seen specialist mental health services in the preceding year (Sayal, Yates, Spears, & Stallard, 2014).

Linking up NHS provision with others such as voluntary sector youth information, advice and counselling services – although critical – can also be a challenge. Any discussion about meeting the need for mental health services among children and young people needs to take into account this wider realm of provision, including the voluntary and independent sectors. These deal with a significant proportion of young people who do not meet the threshold for CAMHS.

Conclusion

Child mental health is a big issue, both in terms of the extent of the difficulties experienced by significant proportions of the child and adolescent population, but also because of the challenges posed in trying to meet need within existing services, both statutory and beyond. Mental health is as significant as physical health in terms of long-term outcomes and impacts on unfolding lives, yet investment in mental health lags a long way behind physical health services. Ensuring we have up-to-date, robust epidemiological data is a critical part of mapping need, planning interventions and tracking time trends.

Summary of key findings

- Mental health disorders are common in children and adolescence, with at least one in 10 experiencing difficulties at any given time.
- Common mental health problems include behaviour disorders, anxiety and depression, and attention deficit and hyperactivity disorders. These can be distinguished from the ordinary ups and downs of childhood or adolescence.
- Formal diagnoses are useful but do not capture all that we know about problems young people face; many reach services with complicated needs for support but without falling neatly into diagnostic criteria.
- A number of different agencies and providers provide interventions and treatment, including both statutory health services but also voluntary sector organizations and others working in schools, the community and primary care.
- There is evidence of a substantial 'treatment gap', with perhaps more than half of those needing treatment not getting it.

Recommended reading

De Los Reyes, A., Augenstein, T., Want, M., Thomas, S., Drabick, D., Burgers, D., & Rabinowitz, J. (2015). The validity of the multi-informant approach to assessing child and adolescent mental health. *Psychological Bulletin*, 141(4), 858–900. A helpful meta-analysis and evaluation of the validity of the multi-informant approach in clinical child and adolescent assessment.

Department of Health. (2015). *Future in mind: Promoting, protecting and improving our children and young people's mental health and wellbeing.* London: DH. Report with recommendations from a taskforce co-chaired by NHS England and the Department of Health, which spells out the situation at the time and includes a number of proposals for improving children and young people's mental health services.

Green, H., McGinnity, A., Meltzer, H., Ford, T., & Goodman, R. (2005). *Mental health of children and young people in Great Britain, 2004.* London: Office for National Statistics. Report of findings from the second (2004) national survey of the mental health of children and young people in Britain.

Goodman, R., & Scott, S. (2012). *Child and adolescent psychiatry* (3rd ed.). Chichester: Wiley-Blackwell. Accessible child and adolescent psychiatry textbook for clinicians, trainees and students, with sections on assessment, individual disorders, risk factors, and treatment/prevention.

Hagell, A., Coleman, J., & Brooks, F. (2015). *Key data on adolescence 2015.* London: Association for Young People's Health. See particularly Chapter 6 on mental health and Chapter 8 on service use. Compendium of publicly available statistics on young people's health, including downloadable spreadsheets containing the original data, and an accompanying set of PowerPoint slides for use in presentations (available on the 'Key Data on Adolescence' page on AYPH's website, www.youngpeopleshealth.org.uk/key-data-on-adolescence).

Jones, P. B. (2013). Adult mental health disorders and their age at onset. *British Journal of Psychiatry*, 202, s5–s10. Review of evidence that many adult mental health disorders begin by adolescence, and discussion of implications for service provision.

Maughan, B., Collishaw, S., & Stringaris, A. (2013). Depression in childhood and adolescence. *Journal of the Canadian Academy of Child and Adolescent Psychiatry*, 22(1), 35–42. Brief review of developmental trends in depressive disorders; patterns of comorbidity; risk factors; and efficacy of current treatment approaches.

Merikangas, K. R., Nakamua, E. R., & Kessler, R. C. (2009). Epidemiology of mental disorders in children and adolescents. *Dialogues in Clinical Neuroscience*, 11(1), 7–20. Review of the rates of mental disorders in children and adolescents from recent community surveys across the world.

National Institute for Health and Clinical Excellence (NICE) (2005). *Depression in children and young people: Identification and management. NICE Guidelines CG20* Retrieved from www.nice.org.uk/guidance/cg28 The NICE guideline on depression in children and young people, covering care pathways, what to expect from treatment, and information on the kinds of services on offer.

Thapar, A., Pine, D., Leckman, J., Scott, S., Snowling, M., & Taylor, E. (Eds.). (2015). *Rutter's child and adolescent psychiatry* (6th ed.). Chichester: Wiley-Blackwell. Comprehensive textbook with sections devoted to conceptual issues and research approaches; influences on psychopathology; approaching the clinical encounter; and clinical syndromes.

Questions for reflection

- How has this chapter helped you to think about the difference between the ordinary ups and downs of adolescence and more formal diagnoses of mental ill health?

(Continued)

(Continued)

- What are the limitations in basing what we know about trends in child mental health on standard diagnostic categories?
- How confident are you that we know what the trends are in young people's mental health? what makes you less confident?

References

American Psychiatric Association (2013). *Diagnostic and statistical manual of mental disorders* (5th ed.). Washington, DC: APA.

Angold, A., & Egger, H. L. (2007). Preschool psychopathology: Lessons for the lifespan. *Journal of Child Psychology and Psychiatry*, 48, 961–966.

Angold, A., Erkanli, A., Copeland, W., Goodman, R., Fisher, P. W., & Costello, E. J. (2012). Psychiatric diagnostic interviews for children and adolescents: A comparative study. *Journal of the American Academy of Child and Adolescent Psychiatry*, 51, 506–517.

Arcelus, J., Mitchell, A., Wales, J., & Nielsen, S. (2011). Mortality rates in patients with anorexia nervosa and other eating disorders. A meta-analysis of 36 studies. *Archives of General Psychiatry*, 68, 724–731.

Bebbington, P. (1996). The origins of sex differences in depressive disorder: Bridging the gap. *International Review of Psychiatry*, 8, 295–332.

Bronfenbrenner, U. (1979). *The ecology of human development: Experiments by nature and design.* Cambridge, MA: Harvard University Press.

Brooks, F., Magnusson, J., Klemera, E., Chester, K., Spencer, N., & Smeeton, N. (2015). *HBSC England national report: Health behaviour in school-aged children: WHO collaborative cross national study.* Hatfield: University of Hertfordshire.

Caspi, A., Houts, R., Belsky, D., Goldman-Mellor, S., Harrington, H., Israel, S., Meier, M., Ramrakha, S., Shalev, I., Roulton, R., & Moffitt, T. (2013). The p factor: One general psychopathology factor in the structure of psychiatric disorders? *Clinical Psychological Science*, 2, 119–137.

Chorpita, B. F., Yim, L., Moffitt, C., Umemoto, L. A., & Francis, S. E. (2000). Assessment of symptoms of DSM-IV anxiety and depression in children: A revised child anxiety and depression scale. *Behaviour Research and Therapy*, 38, 835–855.

Collishaw, S., Maughan, B., Goodman, R., & Pickles, A. (2004). Time trends in adolescent mental health. *Journal of Child Psychology and Psychiatry*, 45, 1350–1362.

De Los Reyes, A., Augenstein, T., Want, M., Thomas, S., Drabick, D., Burgers, D., & Rabinowitz, J. (2015). The validity of the multi-informant approach to assessing child and adolescent mental health. *Psychological Bulletin*, 141, 858–900.

Department of Health. (2015). *Future in mind: Promoting, protecting and improving our children and young people's mental health and wellbeing.* London: DH.

Goodman, R. (1999). The extended version of the Strengths and Difficulties Questionnaire as a guide to child psychiatric caseness and consequent burden. *Journal of Child Psychology and Psychiatry*, 40, 791–799.

Green, H., McGinnity, A., Meltzer, H., Ford, T., & Goodman, R. (2005). *Mental health of children and young people in Great Britain, 2004.* London: Office for National Statistics.

Grills, A. E., & Ollendick, T. H. (2002). Issues in parent–child agreement: The case of structured diagnostic interviews. *Clinical Child and Family Psychology Review*, 5, 57–83.

Hagell, A. (2012). *Changing adolescence: Social trends and mental health.* Bristol: Policy Press.

Hagell, A., Coleman, J., & Brooks, F. (2015). *Key data on adolescence 2015.* London: Association for Young People's Health.

Hawton, K., Saunders K., & O'Connor, R. (2012). Self-harm and suicide in adolescents. *Lancet*, 379, 2373–2382.

Health and Social Care Information Centre (2014). *Provisional monthly hospital episode statistics for admitted care, outpatients and A&E data, April 2013–October 2013: Topic of interest – Eating disorders.* Leeds: HSCIC.

House of Commons Health Committee (2014). *Child and adolescent mental health and CAMHS. Third report of session 2014–15.* London: House of Commons.

Jones, P. B. (2013). Adult mental health disorders and their age at onset. *British Journal of Psychiatry,* 202, s5–s10.

Kessler, R., Bergulund, P., Demler, O., Jin, R., Merikangas, K., & Walters, E. (2005). Lifetime prevalence and age-of-onset distributions of DSM-IV disorders in the National Comorbidity Survey Replication. *Archives of General Psychiatry,* 62, 593–602.

Kim-Cohen, J., Caspi, A., Moffitt, T. E., Harrington, H., Milne, B. J., & Poulton, R. (2003). Prior juvenile diagnoses in adults with mental disorder: Developmental follow-back of a prospective-longitudinal cohort. *Archives of General Psychiatry,* 60, 709–717.

Knapp, M., Ardino, V., Brimblecombe, N., Evans-Lacko, S., Immi, V., King, D., Snell, T., Murguia, S., Mbeah-Bankas, H., Crane, S., Harris, A., Fowler, D., Hodgekins, J., & Wilson, J. (2016). *Youth mental health: New economic evidence.* London: Young Minds and LSE PSSRU.

Maughan, B., Collishaw, S., Meltzer, H., & Goodman, R. (2008). Recent trends in UK child and adolescent mental health. *Social Psychiatry and Psychiatric Epidemiology,* 43, 305–310.

Merikangas, K., He, J., Burstein, M., Swanson, S., Avenevoli, S., Cui, L., Benjet, C., Georgiades, K., & Swendsen, J. (2010). Lifetime prevalence of mental disorders in US adolescents: Results from the National Comorbidity Study – Adolescent Supplement (NCS-A). *Journal of the American Academy of Child and Adolescent Psychiatry,* 49, 980–989.

National Collaborating Centre for Mental Health (2012). *Eating disorders.* Leicester: British Psychological Society.

National Institute for Health and Clinical Excellence (2005). Depression in children and young people: Identification and management. NICE Guidelines CG20. Retrieved from www.nice.org.uk/guidance/cg28

NHS Benchmarking Network (2013). *Raising standards through sharing excellence: CAMHS benchmarking report.* London: NHS BN.

O'Connor, R., Rasmussen, S., Miles, J., & Hawton, K. (2009). Self-harm in adolescents P: Self-report survey in schools in Scotland. *British Journal of Psychiatry,* 194, 68–72.

Pickett, W., Molcho, M., Elgar, F., Brooks, F., de Looze, M., Rathmann, K., et al. (2013). Trends and socioeconomic correlates of adolescent physical fighting in 30 countries. *Pediatrics,* 131, e18–e26.

Rutter, M. (2012). Resilience as a dynamic concept. *Development and Psychopathology,* 24, 335–344.

Rutter, M., Moffitt, T., & Caspi, A. (2006). Gene-environment interplay and psychopathology: Multiple varieties but real effects. *Journal of Child Psychology and Psychiatry,* 47, 226–261.

Sayal, K., Yates, N., Spears, M., & Stallard, P. (2014). Service use in adolescents at risk of depression and self-harm: Prospective longitudinal study. *Social Psychiatry and Psychiatric Epidemiology,* 49, 1231–1240.

Simonoff, E., Pickles, A., Charman, T., Chandler, S., Loucas, T., & Baird, G. (2008). Psychiatric disorders in children with autism spectrum disorders: Prevalence, comorbidity, and associated factors in a population-derived sample. *Journal of the American Academy of Child and Adolescent Psychiatry,* 47, 921–929.

Snell, T., Knapp, M., Healey, A., Gugliani, S., Evans-Lacko, S., Fernandez, J., Meltzer, H., & Ford, T. (2013). Economic impact of childhood psychiatric disorder on public sector services in Britain: estimates from national survey data. *Journal of Child Psychology and Psychiatry,* 54, 977–985.

Thapar, A., Pine, D., Leckman, J., Scott, S., Snowling, M., & Taylor, E. (Eds.). (2015). *Rutter's child and adolescent psychiatry* (6th ed.). Chichester: Wiley-Blackwell.

Van der Ende, J., Verhulst, F., and Tiemeier, H. (2012). Agreement of informants on emotional and behavioural problems from childhood to adulthood. *Psychological Assessment,* 24, 293–300.

Whiteford, H., Degenhardt, L., Rehgm, J., et al. (2013). Global burden of disease attributable to mental and substance use disorders: Findings from the Global Burden of Disease Study. *Lancet,* 382, 1575–1586.

Wolfe, I., Macfarlane, A., Donkin, A., Marmot, M., & Viner, R. (2014). *Why children die: Death in infants, children and young people in the UK Part A.* London: Royal College of Paediatrics and Child Health and National Children's Bureau.

Wolpert, M., Harris, R., Hodges, S., Fuggle, P., James, R., Wiener, A., McKenna, C., Law, D., York, A., Jones, M., & Fonagy, P. (2015). *Thrive elaborated.* London: Evidence Based Practice Unit CAMHS Press.

World Health Organization (2010). *International classification of diseases* (10th ed.). Geneva: WHO.

World Health Organization (2013). *Comprehensive mental health action plan 2013–2020.* Geneva: WHO.

3

NEUROBIOLOGY, ATTACHMENT AND TRAUMA: THE DEVELOPMENT OF MENTAL HEALTH PROBLEMS IN CHILDREN AND YOUNG PEOPLE

GRAHAM MUSIC

This chapter discusses

This chapter will focus on the importance of developmental research for practitioners working with children, addressing the following:

- Recent neuroscience and the impact of early experiences on the developing brain and psyche of the child
- Attachment theory as a paradigm which delivers crucial understandings of child development
- Mentalization, intersubjectivity, and how emotional growth occurs through mind-to-mind contact
- The profound effects of trauma and maltreatment on the brain
- The centrality of emotional regulation, the nervous system and executive functions
- Why diagnostic models such as DSM/ICD often fail maltreated children
- Epigenetic research, and the relative role of genes and environment
- The longer-term effects of early adverse experiences on both psychological and physical health
- The place of social, culture and socio-economic influences
- Possible new directions

Introduction

This chapter will examine some of the latest and more important research findings about children's emotional and brain development, and think about why such research is important for practitioners. Much recent developmental research makes it impossible to deny the powerful formative influences of early experiences, on the brain, on the nervous system and on future life trajectories. This evidence can be used as a basis for arguing for certain types of child therapeutic interventions, and can inform the way that we work. The chapter provides a roadmap to navigate important research findings and pointers from which readers can further explore the issues.

As well as neurobiology, the chapter looks at attachment theory which, although this chapter does not claim is the only theory relevant to child development, nevertheless provides an important lens through which to examine how children develop emotionally, and how expectations and beliefs about relationships develop as responses to specific parenting styles. We see how attachment styles are adaptive and appropriate responses to particular parenting environments. Issues such as developmental trauma (Van der Kolk, 2005), which includes child abuse, neglect and ongoing maltreatment, and disrupted attachment are given more focus than other causes of psychological problems for two reasons. Firstly, they offer a model for understanding the impact of a range of childhood experiences, such as divorce or parental illness; secondly, because children who suffer more early difficulty are much more likely to be affected by these other disruptive life events (Van Niel, Pachter, Wade, Felitti, & Stein, 2014).

One central theme of attachment theory is the predictive quality of parental states of mind, and of their ability to understand the thoughts and feelings of their children. It is this quality of mind-mindedness (Meins, Fernyhough, Wainwright, Gupta, Fradley & Tuckey, 2002), we will see, which is hugely predictive of a range of characterological developments in children, from secure attachment to the ability to regulate emotions. It is the quality of relationships, particularly empathy and emotional understanding, in effect mentalization, that is crucially important, both in parenting and other growth-enhancing relationships.

We also look at the opposite of growth-enhancing experiences, exploring the latest research about the neurobiological effects of trauma, abuse and neglect. We take a whole body approach, looking at the effects of maltreatment not only on the brains but also on the bodies and nervous systems of children. The consequences of bad experiences are becoming clearer, as are the ways that they give rise to a range of typical behavioural effects. However too often in services we see a lack of developmental understanding and a consequent risk of misdiagnosis and mis-labelling of children who have suffered trauma.

What current research makes clear is that genes, on their own, explain very little. So we look at **epigenetic research** which shows that different experiences, literally, turn on or off a range of genetic potentials. In this way, nurture and nature are in constant interaction. The effects of these experiences are seen in children's long-term trajectories. Adverse early experiences affect how genes are expressed, how immune systems respond, and the likelihood of both psychological and physical ill health right up into adulthood. These adverse experiences cannot be explained simply by parenting styles, and we will also focus on social, cultural and socio-economic issues, such as the effects of poverty and inequality. From these areas of research, implications for practice, policy and service development are drawn.

The brain and early development

Neuroplasticity

In recent decades our understanding of our incredibly complex brains has grown hugely. Amazingly the average brain has 100 billion neurons, and 100 trillion synapses. The average neuron connects directly to 10,000 other neurons. A piece of brain the size of a grain of sand contains 100,000 neurons, 2 million axons and a billion synapses. We can think about the brain as a muscle group; some areas are strengthened by exercise while others wither from neglect.

We are born with an overabundance of brain cells and post-natally there is a massive process of 'pruning'. Cells that are not used simply die off, probably as many as 20 billion synapses between childhood and early adolescence (Schwartz and Begley, 2002), although new wiring can still form later in life. New experience is filtered through already-formed pathways, just as water will naturally flow down existing channels. Hence, as 'Hebb's law' (1949) states, 'cells that fire together wire together'. Schore (1994) has added 'and survive together'. Our brain's architecture is thus formed by the kinds of experiences we have.

Box 3.1 Key studies: Parental conflict shapes a baby's brain development

The human brain adapts fast to its environment, and is a powerful predictor (Clark, 2013) of the future. Infants as young as 6 months whose parents reported couple conflict were brought into a lab and placed in fMRI scanners while sleeping (Graham, Fisher, & Pfeifer, 2013). Compared to infants whose parents reported less conflict, these infants showed much higher reactivity in a range of brain regions central to fear when hearing a deep male voice. The brains of these tiny babies were, presumably, quickly adapted to be ready for danger, even in their sleep!

The human brain, and particularly the infant brain, is very malleable, a capacity described as neuroplasticity (Begley, 2009; Doidge, 2008). The period from the last trimester of pregnancy through to the second year of life is crucial. Thankfully, however, some plasticity remains throughout the lifespan, particularly during adolescence.

Triune brain?

Different parts of our complex brains evolved at different stages of our evolutionary history and serve different functions. Although simplified, MacLean's (1990) concept of the triune (three part) brain is a useful starting point (see Figure 3.1). This theory uses the metaphor of the reptilian brain, the limbic system and the most evolutionary advanced neocortex.

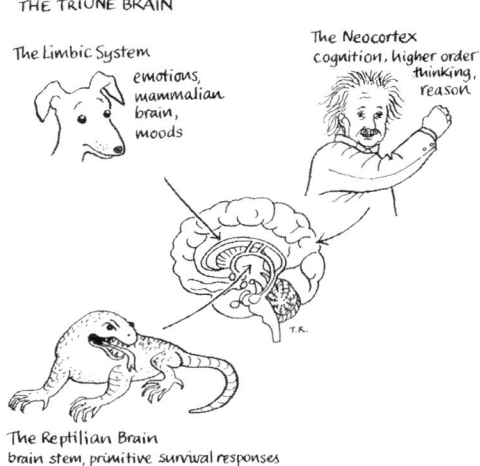

THE TRIUNE BRAIN

The Limbic System
emotions, mammalian brain, moods

The Neocortex
cognition, higher order thinking, reason

The Reptilian Brain
brain stem, primitive survival responses

Figure 3.1   The triune brain

We share much brain functioning with reptiles, such as the areas controlling heart-rate, breathing, temperature and balance, and structures such as the brain stem which are vital for consciousness (Solms and Panksepp, 2012), but also control survival instincts for dominance and aggression.

The limbic system came into existence with mammals and is really the seat of our emotional life. It is concerned with making judgements, learning whether an experience is likely to be pleasurable or not, and forming emotional memories. It contains vital structures such as the amygdala, centrally important for emotions such as fear; and the hippocampus, which has an important role in memory.

The 'new kid on the block' is the neocortex, which includes the frontal lobes. It is a mere 2 or 3 million years old, and its most complex form is seen in humans. Without it there is no thought, language, empathy, executive functions or imagination.

In reality, there are not three separate brain areas, and complex relationships and pathways have developed between them over the millennia. However, the shorthand of the triune brain provides a helpful metaphor for making sense of different brain processes.

Box 3.2   Implications for practice

A self-reflective exercise I quite often undertake with myself when working with clients is to ask whether it is the reptilian or mammalian brains or the cerebral cortex that is active at a particular moment. Basic instinctual responses emanate from the reptilian brain, such as hate, lust and aggression, while powerful defensive strategies of fight and flight are seen in the limbic system. If one is confronted by massive anger or hatred in a child who is in 'fight' mode, it is folly to make an intellectually complex comment that only the cerebral cortex could make sense of, as those more complex parts of the brain are offline at such moments.

Autonomic nervous system bodies

Experiences affect not just brains but whole body processes, and neuroscientists have challenged the idea of brains and minds being separate from bodies (Thompson & Cosmelli, 2011). Our autonomic nervous system is central to bodily regulation, and we use different parts of our brain and nervous system when in different moods or contexts, such as when in a loving environment or under threat. When in danger we tend to become very aroused, and resort to primitive survival responses such as fight or flight, or even freeze. Our whole being and physiology is then geared to the threat, and we see increased heart-rate, sweating, quicker breathing, pupil dilation, feeling cold and inhibited digestion. In fear states we tense up and prepare for trouble, while other bodily functions, such as digestion or immune responses, temporarily go into abeyance, as do higher order thought processes. Some children suffer extreme trauma. By trauma I mean experience that overwhelms the psychological system so that usual coping strategies fail. An experience might be traumatic for one child but might not be another if they have more resilience factors. Some situations would be overwhelming for just about any child, and multiple traumatic experiences over time may give rise to 'disorganized attachment relationships'. Such children are often predisposed into the dysregulated states, described above, very speedily. Such reactions are part of the sympathetic nervous system, which includes the fight–flight response, and is seen in all mammals. These three aspects of the autonomic nervous system are illustrated in Figure 3.2.

We have two main stress response systems, an incredibly fast one, linked to the release of adrenaline, and the HPA (hypothalamic-pituitary-adrenal) axis, involving the stress hormone cortisol, a slower-burning but long-lasting system. We all need

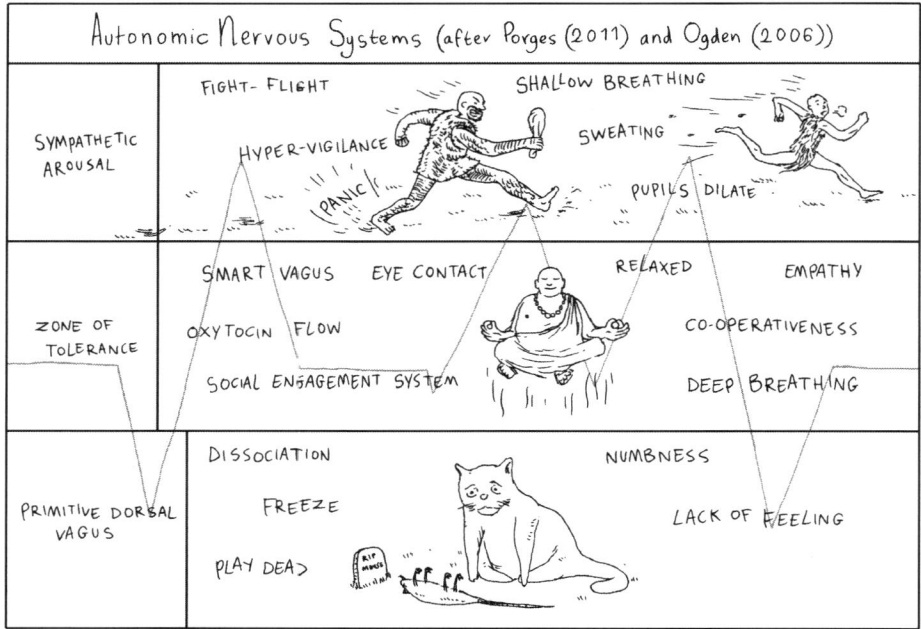

Figure 3.2 The autonomic nervous system

such arousal systems when frightened or angry, but some children get stuck in this way of being.

Box 3.3   Implications for practice

Think of a child who recently acted aggressively or impulsively and try to imagine why they became so aroused, what might be going on to trigger what seems an extreme reaction. Imagine what might be happening in both their mind and body, and try also to think about how this might relate to their early experiences.

Porges (2011) suggests that we have an even more primitive response to terror which we share with the least developed of species and depends on the evolutionarily ancient dorsal vagus nerve. Its activation leads to complete immobilization, freezing and the closing down of our systems. Dissociation and metabolic shutdown are typical of this 'rabbit in the headlights' system. It is adaptive because predators are not attracted to creatures that seem lifeless; but we should worry about children in this state, as they are often not spotted by the adults around them, as they tend to be quiet and not cause trouble, such as perhaps when a family is visited by services and the children seem quiet.

The most advanced element of our autonomic nervous system, from an evolutionary perspective, depends on a sophisticated (ventral) branch of our vagus nerve which connects our brain stem, heart, stomach and facial muscles. This 'smart' vagus is active in bonding, attachment, social communication, empathy and care for others. It turns off when we feel anxious or threatened, has an opposite effect to the sympathetic nervous system's arousing mechanisms and is part of the parasympathetic nervous system which calms us down. It links the brain, heart and stomach, which have their own neurons and nervous systems. While it is seen as a vagal 'brake' that is firing away when we feel good, the vagal brake comes off when we need to move into defensive sympathetic nervous system responses.

Vagal tone is easily measured through how variable our heart-rate is. Variable heart-rates are very predictive of good mental and physical health, better emotional regulation, secure attachment (Diamond, Fagundes, & Butterworth, 2012) and behavioural regulation (Eisenberg, Fabes, Murphy, Karbon, Smith, & Maszk, 1996). It is also a measure that can be used effectively in research. For example, one study found that heart-rate variability improved in clients who were taught self-regulatory skills to manage stressful situations (Cornet, de Kogel, Nijman, Raine, & van der Laan, 2015).

Whole bodies, hormones and opiates

As I have set out above, modern neurobiology takes account of whole bodies, not just brains, and as Damasio (1999) points out, emotions are bodily states. Experiences get written into our body, and one way this happens is via our internal chemical systems and hormones. Traumatized children can become predisposed, for example, to be quickly aroused, releasing large amounts of adrenaline, and the stress hormone, cortisol, in response to the slightest stimulus, such as a loud noise down the road. Such children might not have the buffer of the protective hormones, such as oxytocin, that can lower fear and increase feelings of ease.

The human brain produces many hormones and opiates, some of the best known being cortisol (the 'stress hormone'), dopamine, oxytocin (sometimes called the 'cuddle hormone') as well as endogenous opioids and endorphins. Children starting nursery develop higher levels of cortisol than when they were in home-based care (Groeneveld, Vermeer, van IJzendoorn, & Linting, 2010). Understanding the role that each of these plays, in both a helpful and problematic way, can be useful for clinicians working with children.

Although helpful in the short-term, cortisol has a number of pernicious long-term effects. This leads Gerhardt (2014) to dub it 'corrosive cortisol', particularly in light of how it can attack cells in the hippocampus, the part of the brain that is central to memory. Occasionally extreme trauma can have the opposite effect and result in extremely low cortisol levels – often seen in post-traumatic stress disorder (PTSD) victims such as Holocaust survivors (Yehuda, Engel, Brand, Seckl, Marcus, & Berkowitz, 2005). Either way, too much or too little cortisol is not what the human body was designed for.

Oxytocin is particularly important in attachment and bonding (Zak, 2012), as it induces tranquillity, reduces social fear and pain, and increases empathy. We release it when we have a massage, or are being lovingly touched, and with more oxytocin we become more generous (Morhenn, Park, Piper, & Zak, 2008), have lower blood pressure (Holt-Lunstad, Birmingham, & Light, 2008), and even more attention to the eye-regions of those around us (Guastella et al., 2010). The oxytocin levels of human parents of either gender rise considerably in the months after becoming a parent, and the higher the levels, the more affectionate play we see (Gordon, Zagoory-Sharon, Leckman, & Feldman, 2010), and the more sensitivity to infant cues (Strathearn, Iyengar, Fonagy, & Kim, 2012).

Box 3.4   Key studies: Interesting research with oxytocin

When shown pictures of threatening and scary faces, those given oxytocin beforehand had much less activity in their amygdala, the brain area linked with stress and anger, compared to a control group. This suggests that oxytocin lowers social fear (Kirsch et al., 2005). Fathers given oxytocin intra-nasally not only became more sensitive to their infants, but these infants became more responsive in return (Weisman, Zagoory-Sharon, & Feldman, 2012). Giving oxytocin intra-nasally increases people's willingness to cooperate and heightens altruistic tendencies, as well as the expectation that others will cooperate with them (Israel, Weisel, Ebstein, & Bornstein, 2012). In a classic trust experiment, popularized by Paul Zak, subjects were given either oxytocin or a placebo. All were given money and a choice about whether to give an amount to a stranger who might, but might not, give them up to four times as much back. The oxytocin group were more trusting and generous, gave more away and reaped the rewards as they received more back.

Other neurochemicals also play a central role in attachment and emotional well-being, such as serotonin, targeted by antidepressant drugs and fundamentally linked to feeling good. We see low levels of it in depression, alongside irritability and aggression, both in humans and primates (Carver, Johnson, & Joormann, 2008). Childhood adversity such as maternal depression or trauma gives rise to lower serotonin levels (Field, 2011). Similarly dopamine is central to what Panksepp (Panksepp & Biven, 2012) calls 'seeking' behaviours: wanting things, being excited and hopeful. For example, both depressed mothers and their new-born babies have lower levels of both dopamine and serotonin.

Our hormonal systems can get programmed really early on. Cortisol levels are higher and stress systems more highly activated even in neonates as a result of pre-natal stress and cortisol levels crossing the placenta (Glover, 2014).

Box 3.5   Key studies: Sensitive care affects cortisol levels

Cortisol levels are also easily measurable, such as via saliva swabs, and can be used in research. A good example is in the work of Mary Dozier (Dozier et al., 2006). She researched maltreated children under 18 months who were placed in foster care. Those who were placed with foster carers who were emotionally sensitive and who were catego-rized as secure-autonomous in the Adult Attachment Interview, not only often changed from insecure to secure attachment styles, but their cortisol levels also changed to more healthy levels (Bernard, Dozier, Bick, & Gordon, 2014).

The hormones and chemicals in our bodies are not only responsive to negative expe-riences. Our neurochemicals work as a key and lock system: we need the receptors for them to lock onto to take effect. Experiences partly determine how many recep-tors form, and the more good loving experiences we have early on in life then the more oxytocin receptors we are likely to develop, and so later oxytocin release becomes more effective. However, early stressful life experiences lead to fewer oxy-tocin receptors, and lower oxytocin levels both in men (Opacka-Juffry & Mohiyeddini, 2011), and women abused as children (Heim, Young, Newport, Mletzko, Miller, & Nemesoff, 2008). Powerful bodily programming is happening very early on, and is measurably linked to psychological (LeMoult, Ordaz, Kircanski, Singh, & Gotlib, 2015) and behavioural problems (Kohrt, Hruschka, Kohrt, Carrion, Waldman, & Worthman, 2015). It is valuable for clinicians to be aware of the neurobiological impact of early experience when working with children and young people.

Attachment theory

The origins of attachment theory

Attachment theory, originated by John Bowlby at the Tavistock Clinic in London, is one of the most influential bodies of research about children, providing many research les-sons. Bowlby learnt that infants of many species raised without maternal care were badly scarred and he was one of the first to suggest that children had important emo-tional as well as physical needs (Bowlby, 1969). He had studied young criminals and found that most had suffered separations from parents, as well as inconsistent parenting, violence and neglect. Along with colleagues such as James and Joyce Robertson (see Robertson, 1971) at the Hampstead Child Therapy Clinic (now the Anna Freud Centre), he demonstrated the extraordinary stress young children experience when separated from attachment figures. They showed a common cycle from disbelief, protest, crying and screaming, to later slowly sinking into despairing, cut-off states.

Early attachment theory emphasized the importance of attachment figures as a secure base to return to when anxious, giving confidence to explore, even if it overestimated the importance of mothers over other attachment figures (Hrdy, 2009).

Attachment's second phase: Ainsworth's Strange Situation Test, Crittenden's Dynamic Maturational Model

The next phases of attachment theory increased its range and subtlety, showing how different parenting styles influence children to have different patterns of relating. A fairly simple empirical test gave attachment theory a new scientific rigour. The Strange Situation Test, devised by Ainsworth (1978), built on how infants develop stranger anxiety, swiftly seeking out attachment figures when near an unknown person. This test, a straightforward 20-minute procedure, profoundly altered attachment theory. It particularly looks at how infants respond when their parent leaves the room, and they are left alone with a stranger, and also examines their responses when their mother returns.

While this experiment might seem cruel, and might not get past ethics committees today, it has also been fascinating to see the diversity of reactions infants have. Some cry, scream and crawl towards the door but quickly calm on the mother's return; others seem to barely notice their mothers leaving, and appear not to react when they return to the room; and still others are very preoccupied with their mothers before and after separations and cannot settle. As a result of these distinct reactions Ainsworth categorized the behaviours into three main types: securely attached; and two types of insecure attachment, now mostly called avoidant and ambivalent attachment.

Babies who came to be classified as securely attached were those who cried when their mother left, but who greeted their mother's return with relief, and sometimes delight, and then quickly settled back into a relaxed state. The avoidant infants develop a deactivating strategy, seeming not to notice when their mothers leave, although in fact their physiological stress symptoms increase similarly to securely attached children (Sroufe & Waters, 1977). In ambivalent attachment infants are preoccupied and clingy before their mother even leaves, and on her return they remain vigilant and unsettled, or 'hyperactivated'.

This test has been replicated all over the world. Secure infants have parents who seem sensitive to them, who respond to their distress, and who are consistently available. Generally parents of avoidantly attached children tend not to respond to signals such as crying, and of course there is little point crying if no one notices, or if your attachment figure gets cross when you show that you are upset. Ambivalently attached children tend to have more inconsistent parents, maybe available one moment, and withdrawn or preoccupied the next. Such children explore less, are more clingy, enmeshed, and less at ease. It is important to remember that all these attachment strategies are adaptive ways of staying close to carers.

A more worrying group were later discovered (Hesse & Main, 2000) who had often been subjected to traumatizing parenting and failed to develop a coherent attachment strategy, indeed often acting quite bizarrely. Their parent, who should provide solace or comfort, was often the person causing the distress, such as by being violent. This group was classified by Main as disorganized, and such children are often a cause of concern to professionals as they grow up. Crittenden (1993) would argue that many of these children are caught between strategies, veering for example between avoidance and approach.

Box 3.6   Implications for practice

Think of three children you have had recent contact with. Try to imagine what attachment style they have developed based on how they respond to anxiety-provoking situations. Then try to make sense of why they might have developed their particular relational strategies.

Crittenden, another student of Bowlby, developed a slightly different system of classifying attachment (Crittenden, 2015), which is gaining increasing sway. Crittenden's Dynamic Maturational Model (DMM) disavows the notion that some styles are 'healthier', avoiding words like 'insecure' that have a judgemental flavour. She suggests that throughout the lifespan attachment strategies will change in response to changing contexts, and are nearly always adaptive to a child's environment. The best chance of survival comes from working out how to behave in order to retain closeness to one's attachment figures, whatever their emotional style. Crittenden has added a wealth of complexity to attachment theory that cannot be done justice to here. She describes, for example, children who are compulsive caregivers, or overly compliant, or who show false positive affect, and she has devised a multiple-axial way of conceptualizing complex personality traits, particularly in response to maltreatment.

Attachment's third stage: What's going on inside us?

These attachment styles are represented internally in how the world is experienced, as what Bowlby called internal working models and Crittenden describes as dispositional representations. Children learn a strategy that works with particular adults, such as to limit their expressiveness if a parent cannot bear emotional displays. Such models are not static, and are influenced by new experiences, although new experiences are also 'read' in the light of previous expectations. Attachment security has been linked to a range of mental health issues such as depression and anxiety (Muris, Mayer, & Meesters, 2000).

The next leap forward in attachment theory occurred with the development of the Adult Attachment Interview (AAI), which brought this world of minds and representations centre-stage and led to a host of new research (Main, Kaplan, & Cassady, 1985).

Box 3.7 Key studies: The Adult Attachment Interview

The AAI is a semi-structured interview which takes about an hour to complete. It aims to 'surprise the unconscious', revealing important features of the representational world that relate to attachment. For example, one is asked for five adjectives that describe relationships with both parents, and then to supply some memories which explain these. Other questions include giving examples of when one was upset as a child, or of memories of a first separation. Such questions tend to stir up strong emotional responses. The interview is painstakingly transcribed and analysed. Most revealing is not what actually happened in the childhoods described, but rather the manner in which the questions are answered, and in particular the internal coherence, consistency and reflectiveness of the narrative. This has been shown to be predictive of later child outcomes (Fonagy, Steele, & Steele, 1991).

Adults classified as 'secure-autonomous' develop a coherent story about their lives that takes account of emotional experience of self and other. Such adults are most likely to have securely attached children. Narratives of adults who score 'preoccupied' can be angry in places, confused, with more jumbled sentences, full of detail but low on self-reflection. They are most likely to be parents of children with ambivalent attachments. In a 'dismissing' style we see fairly restricted memories which are often falsely positive, and when they do tell stories about their childhood experiences they often contradict the original rosy picture. Being in touch with emotions, particularly negative emotions, does not come easily to this group. The 'unresolved-disorganized' is the fourth group. Their narratives lack coherence and show poor reasoning and bizarre thinking, and their stories often show up trauma and loss. These are parents who tend to be both 'frightened and frightening' and are most likely to have children classified as disorganized.

Importantly, research on the AAI has shown that what is more predictive than an adult's actual childhood is their ability to reflect on experiences. One is more likely to be secure-autonomous if one has had positive childhood experiences, but it is not inevitable. What makes the difference, even if one has had negative experiences, is the ability to self-reflect and 'make peace' with the past to some extent.

Box 3.8 Attachment styles can change, and symptoms too

Attachment styles can change from insecure to secure with changes in psychological functioning (Dozier et al., 2006). There is growing evidence that psychodynamic psychotherapy can lead to positive changes in children's attachment styles (Stefini, Horn, Winkelmann, Geiser-Elze, Hartmann, & Kronmüller, 2013), as of course can a change in parenting or placement. Other studies have shown that changes in psychotherapy led to lessening of a range of symptoms. For example a study of interpersonal psychotherapy (IPT) with adolescents saw improved social skills, less parental conflict and lower rates of depression alongside more secure attachment styles (Spence, O'Shea, & Donovan, 2015).

Mind-to-mind as central

Children with different attachment styles experience the world differently. Those with a secure attachment style expect positive interactions with others, have the confidence to explore, tend to have more flexibility and capacity to play, more ability to empathize, get on with other children, and regulate their emotions.

While there remains something of a 'transmission gap' (Sette, Coppola, & Cassibba, 2015) in explaining exactly how parental states of mind affect attachment styles, parental sensitivity appears to be central. The concept of 'mind-mindedness' developed by Meins (Meins et al., 2012) in particular predicts whether a child will be securely attached. More mind-minded parents tend to focus on their children's feelings, thoughts and experiences. If a preverbal infant shows distress, the mind-minded parent might speculate aloud about why they are upset, maybe saying 'oh yes you have missed mummy' or 'well that was a frightening loud noise'. Meins showed that repeated experience of one's mental states being reflected upon helps children become aware of both their own and others' mental states. Mothers of avoidantly attached children tend to make relatively few mind-minded comments, whereas mothers of securely attached children make many more, and mothers of ambivalent children might make some mental state statements but these are often an inaccurate reading of the child's internal state.

Thus the ability to understand a child's state of mind is very important. The number of maternal mind-minded comments about a child at 6 months predicts attachment security at a year (Bernier & Dozier, 2003), mentalizing capacities at 48 months (Meins et al., 2003), and both theory of mind as well as verbal and narrative skills at 5 years old (Meins, Fernyhough, Arnott, Leekam, & Rosnay, 2013).

Most developmental research, such as that of Beebe (Beebe, Knoblauch, Rustin, Sorter, Jacobs, & Pally, 2005), Stern (Stern, 1985), Tronick (Tronick, 2007) and countless others, has demonstrated the importance of early attuned parenting, empathy, sensitivity and the ability to 'contain' (Bion, 1962) and process the emotional experiences that children have. A concept with much in common with mind-mindedness that explains much of this is mentalization, developed by Peter Fonagy and others at the Anna Freud Centre (Fonagy, Gyorgy, Jurist, & Target, 2004). This describes the ability to make sense of one's own and others' mental states and to understand how people's behaviour is driven by psychological and emotional factors. A focus on promoting mentalization is increasingly part of treatments for a range of children and young people (Midgley & Vrouva, 2012), but was originally developed for work with adults with borderline personality disorders (Bateman & Fonagy, 2004).

Attachment theory is one perspective from which to understand the ways in which children adapt to their environment, although very early attachment status is not necessarily predictive of longer-term outcomes (Beijersbergen, Juffer, Bakermans-Kranenburg, & van IJzendoorn, 2012). Thankfully, children continue to adapt throughout the lifespan to their current environment and there is less continuity between childhood and adult attachment than one might think, although parental sensitivity at different ages remains a good predictor of security of attachment across the ages (Schoenmaker, Juffer, van Ijzendoorn, Linting, van der Voort, & Bakermans-Kranenburg, 2015). This in turn is a good predictor of some mental health issues, especially disorganized attachment.

Attachment theory and culture

While attachment theory seems to describe a universal biological system, like all theories it is limited by its specific cultural and historical origins. It is certainly possible to apply the concepts and protocols of attachment theory, such as the Strange Situation Test, across cultures, revealing definite cultural variations. For example, the Grossmanns found that in a north German sample avoidant attachment was more common than in south German children (Grossmann, Grossmann, & Waters, 2005). Similarly in Israeli Kibbutz children with communal sleeping arrangements, ambivalent patterns were predominant (Sagi, van Ijzendoorn, Aviezer, Donnell, Koren-Karie, Joels, & Harel, 1995) for children not sleeping with their mothers. Some cultures simply do not seem to have children who fall into certain categories. For example, in the Dogon people in Mali (True, Pisani, & Oumar, 2001), where the mother is the main attachment figure and sleeps with her infants, 87 per cent of the children were categorized as secure, and none at all as avoidant. However, some were disorganized, with mothers who were frightened or frightening.

Attachment categories are relatively broad, which is a strength, as they can be so widely applied, but also a weakness for understanding more subtle nuances. For example, in China, the attachment relationship with paternal grandparents is hugely predictive of a range of outcomes, irrespective of attachment to parents (Liu, 2016). Also, all secure children are not the same. Japanese secure children cry less when leaving their mother's arms than secure German children. Both groups of children have the same secure classification but develop slightly different strategies.

Possibly the very concepts of attachment theory contain cultural biases. Concepts like 'timely responsiveness' or 'maternal sensitivity' have different meanings across cultures. Rothbaum and Morelli (2005) suggest a cultural bias in how attachment theory values autonomy, exploration and independence – capacities more prized in the West. Puerto Rican mothers, for example, tend to be more concerned with calm, respectful attentiveness than autonomy. Physical control of children might be associated with insecurity in American families but with security in Puerto Rican families (Carlson and Harwood, 2003). Similarly, maternal interference predicts attachment insecurity in America but not in Colombia where the opposite is true (Posada & Jacobs, 2001).

Nonetheless, there is compelling evidence for a universal attachment system in human infants, and evidence from cultures as unrelated as Colombia, Mali, Chile and others suggests that parental sensitivity is linked to attachment security, with scores being examined by raters from different cultures. It is true, as Keller (2013) argues, that attachment theory has sometimes failed to recognize the importance of cultural differences and some of its emphases, such as on the role of mothers, or on the importance of autonomy, are less central in some cultures compared to others. Despite this, generally attachment theory appears to retain significant applicability across cultures.

Box 3.9   Gaps in research and implications for practice

A gap in the research is the extent to which cultural biases can inform therapeutic interventions which are alien to a client's cultural beliefs.

A practice example is a therapist who suggested to a parent that she was being intrusive when massaging her child, whereas in fact this act was seen as good parenting in the culture this mother was from. Try to think about an example where your assumptions about what is good parenting might be partly a result of your cultural prejudice.

Long-term effects of early experiences

The previous section looked at attachment and some of the precursors of later psychological issues. This section looks at some longer-term consequences of early experiences, particularly of serious maltreatment. What the research shows is that the worse the early experiences, the poorer the outcomes, and this can be described in terms of neurobiological development.

Brains again

A whole host of research is combining to show that trauma and abuse and early levels of stress affect a range of brain areas (Andersen & Teicher, 2008) (Figure 3.3 shows areas of the brain). Victims of trauma and abuse have a smaller corpus callosum, which links left and right hemispheres, with fewer nerve endings, and so less capacity both for the hemispheres to communicate effectively, and to work better in tandem (Teicher, Dumont, Ito, Vaituzis, Giedd, & Andersen, 2004). We also know that there is much higher activation of the amygdala, central to processing fear and other strong emotions, in those subjected to trauma and violence, leading them to be far more reactive and less able to be still and calm (Sigurdsson, Doyère, Cain, & LeDoux, 2007; Thomas et al., 2001). For example, traumatized children tend to spot anger much more quickly than other children, and emotionally reactive brain areas such as the amygdala fire up much more powerfully (McCrory, De Brito, & Viding, 2010). In children adopted from very neglectful backgrounds,

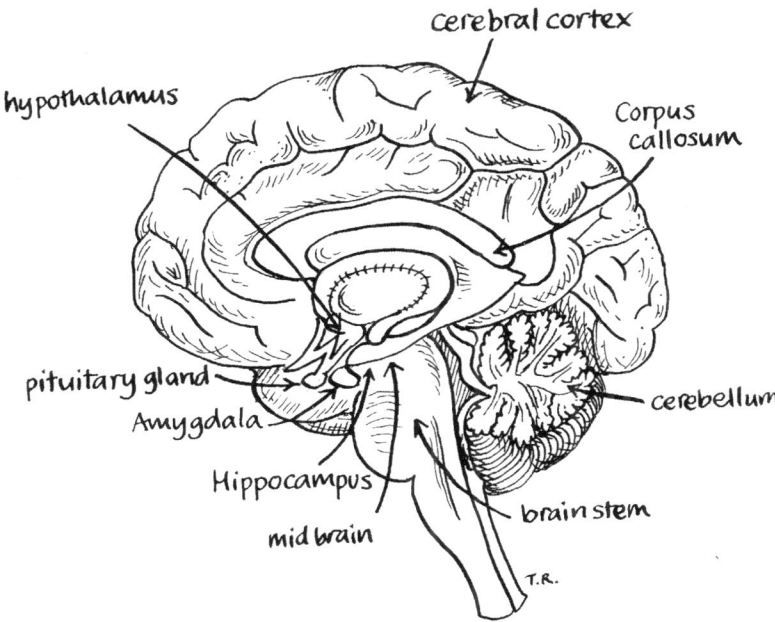

Figure 3.3   The areas of the brain

on the other hand, there is less amygdala activation when witnessing anger or other high levels of emotion. This, again, was presumably adaptive, as such children needed to turn away from an interest in other people's thoughts and feelings and find a way to regulate their own emotions (Strathearn, 2011).

Similarly, childhood trauma is linked with smaller hippocampi in adulthood (Andersen, Tomada, Vincow, Valente, Polcari, & Teicher, 2008), and the hippocampus is central to forming and retrieving memories, among other things. We also consistently see less activation of areas in the prefrontal cortex in children who have suffered trauma and abuse as well as severe neglect (Mehta et al., 2009). These prefrontal areas are vital for capacities such as empathy, but also for emotional regulation. Low empathy and an inability to manage emotional stimuli are behind a lot of the problems maltreated children have in being able to manage the kinds of ordinary life experiences that luckier children take in their stride. While there remains a lot more to find out about, what the research is clearly showing, even if still in rudimentary form, is that different experiences give rise to very different forms of brain development.

Neuroception

The more adverse early experiences a child suffers, the more likelihood of poor mental and physical health, and indeed of early death from a range of causes (Felitti & Anda, 2010). We have learnt that early stress particularly has a profoundly negative effect on later psychological and health outcomes (Bazacliu, Loria, Murdison, & Pollock, 2011). We also know that whatever a child's resilience factors, good early parenting leading to secure attachments will act as an inoculation against a biological predisposition to react badly to stress, even when living in poverty (Conradt, Measelle, & Ablow, 2013). Indeed, good experiences and positive emotionality can decrease stress responses (Pressman, Black, & Segerstrom, 2012), as can interventions like mindfulness (Epel, Daubenmier, Moskowitz, Folkman, & Blackburn, 2009), even slowing the ageing process.

Early stress and trauma are particularly linked with what are called metabolic syndrome diseases, such as heart disease, strokes and diabetes (Felitti et al., 1998). A highly stressed life is also linked with a central tell-tale sign of physical ill health and risk of early death, shorter telomeres (Epel et al., 2004), which are caps at the end of each strand of DNA that protects our chromosomes. Short telomeres are a sign of ill health. There appears to be a dose-related response, so that the more the stress, the bigger effect on telomere length and the more likelihood of all kinds of diseases, from cancer to diabetes to heart disease (Price, Kao, Burgers, Carpenter, & Tyrka, 2012). Indeed, one study even found that stress in intrauterine life gave rise to shortened telomeres right up until adulthood (Entringer et al., 2011). Research is showing that when people are anxious, stressed or traumatized we see a speeding up of metabolic processes. One **longitudinal study** showed clearly that the degree of stress people experience, and their response to it (for example, cortisol levels), was predictive of their health outcomes some 10 years later (Almeida, Piazza, Stawski, & Klein, 2011).

Social factors, poverty and inequality

It is important that parents, particularly mothers, are not 'blamed' for poor mental health. Causes are always multifactored. Living in poverty in a run-down or violence-infused neighbourhood has a profound effect on one's ability to parent.

One very interesting study (Griskevicius et al., 2013) showed that children born into worse economic circumstances are likely to have a different psychological makeup through their lifespans. Research based on life history theory, propounded by many evolutionary psychologists (Moule, Decker, & Pyrooz, 2013), seems to be showing that if we are born into an environment where stress, anxiety, fear or trauma are likely, then we live a 'faster life course', and for example, breed earlier (Belsky, Houts, & Fearon, 2010), take more risks, have worse health and also die younger.

Griskevicius, Tybur, Delton and Robertson (2011), for example, found that those born in poorer circumstances took more risks and were more impulsive when faced with the same choices as those who came from safer, more affluent backgrounds. They also had far more signs of stress as measured by various biomarkers such as inflammation and cellular damage. A faster life course has also been shown to be correlated with increased criminality (Moule et al., 2013) as well as predisposing to all manner of health problems, such as asthma (Sampson et al., 2013).

Box 3.10   Life, history, theory

Evolutionary theorists suggest that it makes sense to develop more impulsive, risk-taking strategies if life is expected to be dangerous or short. For example in a very dangerous uncertain world, early puberty and sexual activity, and having more children but investing less in each, might be a better strategy to ensure some genes are passed on. A recent study in America found just this. A harsh environment linked to risk-taking, substance use and promiscuity in girls (Hampson, Andrews, Barckley, Gerrard, & Gibbons, 2016).

Thus, these outcomes cannot be laid at the door of parents only. Via the neuroception process, humans non-consciously read the current environment and react accordingly. Threat can be picked up out of consciousness, such as violence and signs of environmental poverty. For example, in busy cities our metabolism speeds up (Levine, Reysen, & Ganz, 2008), while just living in a deprived area, such as with many boarded up shops, has an effect on body states such as increasing testosterone levels (linked to aggression) in boys (Tarter et al., 2009).

We do of course need good psychological early intervention, and research about the hidden costs of psychosocial stressors should function as a warning that it will never be enough to just try to build resilience factors in individuals and not worry about the effect of poverty and other serious stressors such as violent or degraded neighbourhoods (Karb, Elliott, Dowd, & Morenoff, 2012). Children at social risk who also have high personal resources, in fact, tend to do worse than economically advantaged children with fewer personal resilience factors (Sameroff, Gutman, & Peck, 2003). Poverty, inequality (Wilkinson & Pickett, 2009) and psychosocial stress, particularly within an unequal society, have serious effects.

Box 3.11   Implications for practice: Levels of intervention

Research points us to consider a range of points of intervention. We might offer support to parents, to individual children, to whole families, but also intervene on a community level, in schools or even at a whole macro-society level, each site of intervention having powerful potential outcomes. For example in the Abecedarian Project in Carolina high-risk infants were given interventions in subjects such as language, reading and maths, with a number of hopeful results. The intervention group were more likely to get through higher education, had higher IQ scores right into adulthood, had children later and generally the effects lasted longer than in other programmes. The children who gained the most were the ones who started off most at risk, with less good quality input at home (Campbell et al., 2012).

Genes, environment, epigenetics

A question is often asked about the relative importance of nature and nurture (Music, 2010). Epigenetics, the study of how genetic traits are turned on and off by particular experiences, has found that while our genetic inheritance makes a difference, these genes might either be turned on, or silenced, by particular kinds of experiences. This process of genes being turned on or off is called methylation (or de-methylation).

Importantly what this means is that some children are less badly affected than others by the same abusive experiences. This is called the 'differential susceptibility to rearing hypothesis' (Belsky, 2005). For example, if one has one of two versions of a dopamine receptor gene and has adverse early experiences, then one's outcomes (for example, mental health problems or increased risk-taking) are likely to be worse (Bakermans-Kranenburg & van IJzendoorn, 2011).

Box 3.12   Gaps in research: Genes and treatment

What might be the implications for treatment outcomes of having some genetic variants as opposed to others? Some children, often labelled as 'orchids', benefit more from positive interventions (Bakermans-Kranenburg & van IJzendoorn, 2015), and are also more affected by bad experiences than the so-called 'dandelions' who thrive in any soil (Kennedy, 2013). Might treatment planning take account of children's genetic inheritance? If so, for what genes and for what treatments and how can this be researched?

Some genes, such as the one linked with oxytocin, seemingly affect attachment status, possibly explaining why children may have different responses to the same kinds of parenting (Raby, Cicchetti, Carlson, Cutuli, Englund, & Egeland, 2012). In terms of attachment, the evidence for genes influencing a child's attachment status is much weaker (Prior & Glaser, 2006). Parental sensitivity remains the best predictor of whether a child will be secure or insecure, even if there might be some link between temperament and disorganized attachment (Spangler, 2013).

What seems increasingly clear from recent epigenetic research is that some children are, for genetic reasons, more likely to be affected by both good and bad experiences (Belsky & Hartman, 2014). Nonetheless, despite exciting new research on genes and temperament, parental sensitivity and mind-mindedness remain as good a predictor as we have as yet of the psychological health as well as the attachment status of a child.

Research and issues of diagnosis for children who have experienced trauma and abuse

Despite often purportedly embracing **'evidence-based practice'**, child and adolescent mental health services (CAMHS) often do not have a good enough understanding of children who have suffered abuse or neglect (DeJong, 2010). Many services insist on a diagnosable mental health disorder as a passport of entry. As various reports have found (for example, Luke, Sinclair, Woolgar, & Sebba, 2014), children with an early history of abuse or neglect often do not fit current diagnostic categories and can thus be either excluded from services, or given diagnoses that do not really fit, as even government reports note (DOH and DCCF, 2009). They can also end up with diagnoses that do not really fit them, such as attention deficit and hyperactivity disorder (ADHD) or autism spectrum disorder, as well as conduct disorders (DeJong, 2010; Prior & Glaser, 2006; Tarren-Sweeney, 2010). Another psychiatric category often confused with attachment theory is attachment disorder which, unlike disorganized attachment, is not a research category. Attachment disorder began as an official psychiatric classification describing children who have been chronically neglected. Again, clinicians and researchers have argued that these categories lack a developmental understanding based in research and many lobbied unsuccessfully for a new category, developmental trauma disorder (Van der Kolk, 2005) to be included in DSM-5. These issues have been particularly highlighted in research by Tarren-Sweeney (2013), whose team have been developing measures that more accurately capture the psychological worlds of maltreated children. This enables a more realistic formulation of many attachment- and trauma-related issues that do not get picked up by ICD or DSM classifications. Other research has backed up how many maltreated are wrongly ascribed either autistic spectrum or attachment disorder diagnoses which can be better explained by a child's developmental history of neglect or abuse (McCullough, Stedmon, & Dallos, 2014).

Many psychological and brain studies show that having a traumatic childhood is highly predictive of being impulsive, dysregulated, having poor executive functioning and even of later drug dependence (Ersche, Turton, Chamberlain, Müller, Bullmore, & Robbins, 2012). In families where high levels of negativity, anger or aggression are common, then not surprisingly children tend to struggle much more with emotional regulation (Morris, Silk, Steinberg, Myers, & Robinson, 2007). Where there is violence and aggression we see extreme sympathetic nervous system arousal and many more externalizing behaviours (El-Sheikh, Kouros, Erath, Cummings, Keller, & Staton, 2009). So many of the children I have worked with who have suffered abuse just cannot bear to wait, are far too easily frustrated, and also quickly feel provoked, seeing aggression and threat where others do not. They are likely to then be diagnosed with a disorder such as ADHD, when the real reason for their behaviour is probably due to trauma.

Many traumatized children displaying such behaviours show poor executive functioning, hyperactivity and seem very like children diagnosed with ADHD (DeJong, 2010). They can be out of control but also become increasingly controlling as they grow older. The world for them is frightening and not to be trusted, and the unexpected is rarely something to look forward to, and so they try to avoid change and control events as much as possible.

Box 3.13   Gap in research: Misdiagnosis in clinical populations

Many children receive ADHD or autistic spectrum diagnoses who have experienced trauma or neglect. Aspects of their behaviour are explainable in terms of the kinds of experiences they have received. A gap in the research is to examine clinical samples with such diagnoses and try to unpick which other factors might have led to the symptomatology that has led to the particular diagnosis.

Not all insecurely attached children have a bad prognosis, but disorganized attachment in a one year old baby is a good predictor of psychopathology at 17 years old (Sroufe, 2005). Disorganized attachment often occurs alongside other risk factors for poor mental health outcomes, such as poverty, single parenthood, violence, drug and alcohol use, and poor neighbourhoods. The disorganized child is likely to suffer from high stress levels, a hyper-alert way of being; show 'helpless' and/or 'hostile' behaviours, and the care they receive is often inconsistent, confusing, frightening and leaves them feeling dysregulated. Such children fail to find a strategy to cope, as both approach and withdrawal can induce fear.

Such children often have to deactivate attachment behaviours to survive, cutting themselves off from what is going on inside them, using extreme defences, such as flight, fight or dissociation. They often show jumpy thought processes, and struggle to stay consistently on a single mental track, something often also seen in their parents' confused reports in the AAI. They can struggle cognitively, in relationships, in regulating emotions and in developing consistent interpersonal strategies. Many fail at school, and advance along worrying trajectories, such as into the criminal justice system, psychiatric, or other services.

Conclusion

This chapter has demonstrated how a range of recent research from the fields of developmental psychology, neurobiology, attachment theory and epigenetics has cast important light on our understanding of children's development. Much of this research signposts those working with children to studies which help make sense of the children they are working with, as well as providing ideas for issues that might be further researched. The research also has implications for the way we offer support to children and young people.

Summary of key findings

- A child's brain is profoundly affected by the kinds of early experiences they have.
- Children develop different attachment styles, which are generally appropriate adaptations to the care-giving environments, but may not always serve them well in terms of their later development.
- Early abuse and neglect have a profound effect on the developing brain and nervous system.
- Adverse early experiences have very serious long-term effects on mental and physical health.
- Child maltreatment has been linked to a range of later mental health outcomes, such as depression (MacMillan et al., 2001), anxiety, conduct disorders and criminality (Hoeve, Colins, Mulder, Loeber, Stams, & Vermeiren, 2015), substance misuse (Anda et al., 2002), and a host of psychiatric issues right into adulthood (Mills, Scott, Alati, O'Callaghan, Najman, & Strathearn, 2013).
- The effects of early maltreatment on a child's behaviours and psychological states can be missed in some psychiatric diagnoses.
- Genes and environment interact and some children are more susceptible to good and bad experiences than others.

Recommended reading

DeJong, M. (2010). Some reflections on the use of psychiatric diagnosis in the looked after or 'in care' child population. *Clinical Child Psychology and Psychiatry*, 15, 589–599. This paper examines how the diagnostic system might do a disservice to maltreated children.

Midgley, N., & Vrouva., I. (Eds.). (2012). *Minding the child: Mentalization-based interventions with children, young people and their families.* London: Routledge. A very good introduction to mentalization in relation to children.

Music, G. (2016). *Nurturing natures: Attachment and children's emotional, social and brain development* (2nd ed.). London: Psychology Press. A solid primer covering many aspects of how children develop psychologically.

Prior, V., & Glaser, D. (2006). *Understanding attachment and attachment disorders: Theory, evidence and practice.* London: Jessica Kingsley. A good text covering the important features of attachment theory and research about it.

Schore, A. N. (2012). *The science of the art of psychotherapy.* New York: Norton. An interesting book on the links between psychotherapy and neuroscience.

Questions for reflection

- How might the ideas from attachment theory presented in this chapter help you make sense of a child you are currently working with?
- How does the research described in this chapter influence the way you might think about a child who is seen as 'naughty' or 'badly behaved'?
- Think of a child who you are working with and then imagine at what level an intervention might be most effective (for example, with the child, the whole family, the parents, school, the local community).
- Develop an idea for a research study of your own, using some of the research ideas in this chapter. Think about some of the gaps in research that have been highlighted in this chapter. What kind of research do you think would be important at this stage? How do you think this research could be conducted?

References

Ainsworth, M. D. S. (1978). *Patterns of attachment: A psychological study of the strange situation.* Mahwah, NJ: Lawrence Erlbaum.

Almeida, D. M., Piazza, J. R., Stawski, R. S., & Klein, L. C. (2011). The speedometer of life: Stress, health, and aging. In K. W. Schaie & S. L. Willis (Eds.), *Handbook of the psychology of aging* (7th ed.) (pp. 191–206). San Diego, CA: Academic Press.

Anda, R. F., Whitfield, C. L., Felitti, V. J., Chapman, D., Edwards, V. J., Dube, S. R., & Williamson, D. F. (2002). Adverse childhood experiences, alcoholic parents, and later risk of alcoholism and depression. *Psychiatric Services*, 53, 1001–1009.

Andersen, S., Tomada, A., Vincow, E., Valente, E., Polcari, A., & Teicher, M. (2008). Preliminary evidence for sensitive periods in the effect of childhood sexual abuse on regional brain development. *Journal of Neuropsychiatry and Clinical Neurosciences*, 20, 292–301.

Andersen, S. L., & Teicher, M. H. (2008). Stress, sensitive periods and maturational events in adolescent depression. *Trends in Neuroscience*, 31, 183–191.

Bakermans-Kranenburg, M. J., & van IJzendoorn, M. H. (2011). Differential susceptibility to rearing environment depending on dopamine-related genes: New evidence and a meta-analysis. *Development and Psychopathology*, 23, 39–52.

Bakermans-Kranenburg, M. J., & van IJzendoorn, M. H. (2015). The hidden efficacy of interventions: Gene×environment experiments from a differential susceptibility perspective. *Annual Review of Psychology*, 66, 381–409.

Bateman, A., & Fonagy, P. (2004). *Psychotherapy for borderline personality disorder: Mentalization-based treatment.* New York: Oxford University Press.

Bazacliu, C., Loria, A. S., Murdison, K. A., & Pollock, J. S. (2011). Early life stress decreases diastolic function in angiotensin II sensitized rats. *Journal of Investigative Medicine*, 55, 494–499.

Beebe, B., Knoblauch, S., Rustin, J., Sorter, D., Jacobs, T. J., & Pally, R. (2005). *Forms of intersubjectivity in infant research and adult treatment.* New York: Other Press LLC.

Begley, S. (2009). *The plastic mind.* London: Constable.

Beijersbergen, M. D., Juffer, F., Bakermans-Kranenburg, M. J., & van IJzendoorn, M. H. (2012). Remaining or becoming secure: Parental sensitive support predicts attachment continuity from infancy to adolescence in a longitudinal adoption study. *Development and Psychopathology*, 48, 1277–1282.

Belsky, J. (2005). Differential susceptibility to rearing influence. In B. Ellis & D. Bjorklund (Eds.), *Origins of the social mind: Evolutionary psychology and child development* (pp. 139–163). New York: Guilford Press.

Belsky, J., & Hartman, S. (2014). Gene-environment interaction in evolutionary perspective: Differential susceptibility to environmental influences. *World Psychiatry*, 13, 87–89.

Belsky, J., Houts, R. M., & Fearon, R. M. P. (2010). Infant attachment security and the timing of puberty testing an evolutionary hypothesis. *Psychological Science*, 21, 1195–1201.

Bernard, K., Dozier, M., Bick, J., & Gordon, M. K. (2014). Intervening to enhance cortisol regulation among children at risk for neglect: Results of a randomized clinical trial. *Developmental Psychology*. Online First.

Bernier, A., & Dozier, M. (2003). Bridging the attachment transmission gap: The role of maternal mind-mindedness. *International Journal of Behavioral Development*, 27, 355–365.

Bion, W. R. (1962). *Learning from experience*. London: Heinemann.

Bowlby, J. (1969). *Attachment and loss. Vol. 1, Attachment*. London: Hogarth.

Campbell, F. A., Pungello, E. P., Burchinal, M., Kainz, K., Pan, Y., Wasik, B. H., Barbarin, O. A., Sparling, J. J., & Ramey, C. T. (2012). Adult outcomes as a function of an early childhood educational program: An Abecedarian Project follow-up. *Developmental Psychology*, 48, 1033–1043.

Carlson, V. J., & Harwood, R. L. (2003). Attachment, culture, and the caregiving system: The cultural patterning of everyday experiences among Anglo and Puerto Rican mother–infant pairs. *Infant Mental Health Journal*, 24, 53–73.

Carver, C. S., Johnson, S. L., & Joormann, J. (2008). Serotonergic function, two-mode models of self-regulation, and vulnerability to depression: What depression has in common with impulsive aggression. *Psychological Bulletin*, 134, 912–943.

Clark, A. (2013). Whatever next? Predictive brains, situated agents, and the future of cognitive science. *Behavioral and Brain Sciences*, 36, 181–204.

Conradt, E., Measelle, J., & Ablow, J. C. (2013). Poverty, problem behavior, and promise: Differential susceptibility among infants reared in poverty. *Psychological Science*, 24, 235–242.

Cornet, L. J. M., de Kogel, C. H., Nijman, H. L. I., Raine, A., & van der Laan, P. H. (2015). Neurobiological changes after intervention in individuals with anti-social behaviour: A literature review. *Criminal Behaviour* and *Mental Health*, 25, 10–27.

Crittenden, P. M. (1993). Characteristics of neglectful parents: An information processing approach. *Criminal Justice and Behavior*, 20, 27–48.

Crittenden, P. M. (2015). *Raising parents: Attachment, representation, and treatment*. Oxford: Routledge.

Damasio, A. (1999). *The feeling of what happens: Body and emotion in the making of consciousness* (p. 386). New York: Harcourt Brace.

DeJong, M. (2010). Some reflections on the use of psychiatric diagnosis in the looked after or 'in care' child population. *Clinical Child Psychology and Psychiatry*, 15, 589–599.

Diamond, L. M., Fagundes, C. P., & Butterworth, M. R. (2012). Attachment style, vagal tone, and empathy during mother–adolescent interactions. *Journal of Research on Adolescence*, 22, 165–184.

DOH & DCCF (2009). *Statutory guidance on promoting the health and well-being of looked after children*. Nottingham: Department of Health, Department for Children, Schools and Families.

Doidge, N. (2008). *The brain that changes itself: Stories of personal triumph from the frontiers of brain science*. London: Penguin.

Dozier, M., Peloso, E., Lindhiem, O., Gordon, M. K., Manni, M., Sepulveda, S., Ackerman, J., Bernier, A., & Levine, S. (2006). Developing evidence-based interventions for foster children: An example of a randomized clinical trial with infants and toddlers. *Journal of Social Issues*, 62, 767–785.

Eisenberg, N., Fabes, R. A., Murphy, B., Karbon, M., Smith, M., & Maszk, P. (1996). The relations of children's dispositional empathy-related responding to their emotionality, regulation, and social functioning. *Developmental Psychology*, 32, 195–209.

El-Sheikh, M., Kouros, C. D., Erath, S., Cummings, E. M., Keller, P., & Staton, L. (2009). Marital conflict and children's externalizing behavior: Pathways involving interactions between parasympathetic and sympathetic nervous system activity. *Monographs of the Society for Research in Child Development*, 74, vii–79.

Entringer, S., Epel, E. S., Kumsta, R., Lin, J., Hellhammer, D. H., Blackburn, E. H., Wüst, S., & Wadhwa, P. D. (2011). Stress exposure in intrauterine life is associated with shorter telomere length in young adulthood. *Proceedings of the National Academy of Sciences*, 108, E513–E518.

Epel, E. S., Blackburn, E. H., Lin, J., Dhabhar, F. S., Adler, N. E., Morrow, J. D., & Cawthon, R. M. (2004). Accelerated telomere shortening in response to life stress. *Proceedings of the National Academy of Sciences*, 101, 17312–17315.

Epel, E., Daubenmier, J., Moskowitz, J. T., Folkman, S., & Blackburn, E. (2009). Can meditation slow rate of cellular aging? Cognitive stress, mindfulness, and telomeres. *Annals of the New York Academy of Sciences*, 1172, 34–53.

Ersche, K. D., Turton, A. J., Chamberlain, S. R., Müller, U., Bullmore, E. T., & Robbins, T. W. (2012). Cognitive dysfunction and anxious-impulsive personality traits are endophenotypes for drug dependence. *American Journal of Psychiatry*, 169, 926–936.

Felitti, V. J., & Anda, R. F. (2010). The relationship of adverse childhood experiences to adult medical disease, psychiatric disorders and sexual behavior: Implications for healthcare. In R. A. Lanius, E. Vermetten & C. Pain (Eds.), *The impact of early life trauma on health and disease: The hidden epidemic* (pp. 77–88). Cambridge: Cambridge University Press.

Felitti, V. J., Anda, R. F., Nordenberg, D., Williamson, D. F., Spitz, A. M., Edwards, V., Koss, M. P., & Marks, J. S. (1998). Relationship of childhood abuse and household dysfunction to many of the leading causes of death in adults: The Adverse Childhood Experiences (ACE) Study. *American Journal of Preventive Medicine*, 14, 245–258.

Field, T. (2011). Prenatal depression effects on early development: A review. *Infant Behavior and Development*, 34, 1–14.

Fonagy, P., Gyorgy, G., Jurist, E. L., & Target, M. (2004). *Affect regulation, mentalization, and the development of the self.* London: Karnac Books.

Fonagy, P., Steele, H., & Steele, M. (1991). Maternal representations of attachment during pregnancy predict the organization of infant–mother attachment at one year of age. *Child Development*, 62, 891–905.

Gerhardt, S. (2014). *Why love matters: How affection shapes a baby's brain.* Oxford: Routledge.

Glover, V. (2014). Maternal depression, anxiety and stress during pregnancy and child outcome: What needs to be done. *Best Practice and Research: Clinical Obstetrics and Gynaecology, Perinatal Mental Health: Guidance for the Obstetrician-Gynaecologist*, 28, 25–35.

Gordon, I., Zagoory-Sharon, O., Leckman, J. F., & Feldman, R. (2010). Oxytocin and the development of parenting in humans. *Biological Psychiatry*, 68, 377–382.

Graham, A. M., Fisher, P. A., & Pfeifer, J. H. (2013). What sleeping babies hear: A functional MRI study of interparental conflict and infants' emotion processing. *Psychological Science*, 24, 782–789.

Griskevicius, V., Ackerman, J. M., Cantú, S. M., Delton, A. W., Robertson, T. E., Simpson, J. A., Thompson, M. E., & Tybur, J. M. (2013). When the economy falters, do people spend or save? Responses to resource scarcity depend on childhood environments. *Psychological Science*, 24, 197–205.

Griskevicius, V., Tybur, J. M., Delton, A. W., & Robertson, T. E. (2011). The influence of mortality and socioeconomic status on risk and delayed rewards: A life history theory approach. *Journal of Personality and Social Psychology*, 100, 1015–1026.

Groeneveld, M. G., Vermeer, H. J., van IJzendoorn, M. H., & Linting, M. (2010). Children's wellbeing and cortisol levels in home-based and center-based childcare. *Early Childhood Research Quarterly*, 25, 502–514.

Grossmann, K. E., Grossmann, K., & Waters, E. (Eds.). (2005). *Attachment from infancy to adulthood: The major longitudinal studies.* New York: Guilford Press.

Guastella, A. J., Einfeld, S. L., Gray, K. M., Rinehart, N. J., Tonge, B. J., Lambert, T. J., & Hickie, I. B. (2010). Intranasal oxytocin improves emotion recognition for youth with autism spectrum disorders. *Biological Psychiatry*, 67, 692–694.

Hampson, S. E., Andrews, J. A., Barckley, M., Gerrard, M., & Gibbons, F. X. (2016). Harsh environments, life history strategies, and adjustment: A longitudinal study of Oregon youth. *Personality and Individual Differences*, 88, 120–124.

Hebb, D. O. (1949). *The organisation of behaviour.* New York: Wiley.

Heim, C., Young, L. J., Newport, D. J., Mletzko, T., Miller, A. H., & Nemeroff, C. B. (2008). Lower CSF oxytocin concentrations in women with a history of childhood abuse. *Molecular Psychiatry*, 14, 954–958.

Hesse, E., & Main, M. (2000). Disorganized infant, child, and adult attachment: Collapse in behavioral and attentional strategies. *Journal of the American Psychoanalytic Association*, 48, 1097–1127.

Hoeve, M., Colins, O. F., Mulder, E. A., Loeber, R., Stams, G. J. J. M., & Vermeiren, R. R. J. M. (2015). The association between childhood maltreatment, mental health problems, and aggression in justice-involved boys. *Aggressive Behavior*, 41, 488–501.

Holt-Lunstad, J., Birmingham, W. A., & Light, K. C. (2008). Influence of a 'warm touch' support enhancement intervention among married couples on ambulatory blood pressure, oxytocin, alpha amylase, and cortisol. *Psychosomatic Medicine*, 70, 976–985.

Hrdy, S. B. (2009). *Mothers and others: the evolutionary origins of mutual understanding.* Cambridge, MA: Harvard University Press.

Israel, S., Weisel, O., Ebstein, R. P., & Bornstein, G. (2012). Oxytocin, but not vasopressin, increases both parochial and universal altruism. *Psychoneuroendocrinology*, 37, 1341–1344.

Karb, R. A., Elliott, M. R., Dowd, J. B., & Morenoff, J. D. (2012). Neighborhood-level stressors, social support, and diurnal patterns of cortisol: The Chicago Community Adult Health Study. *Social Science and Medicine*, 75, 1038–1047.

Keller, H. (2013). Attachment and culture. *Journal of Cross-Cultural Psychology*, 44, 175–194.

Kennedy, E. (2013). Orchids and dandelions: How some children are more susceptible to environmental influences for better or worse and the implications for child development. *Clinical Child Psychology and Psychiatry*, 18, 319–321.

Kirsch, P., Esslinger, C., Chen, Q., Mier, D., Lis, S., Siddhanti, S., Gruppe, H., Mattay, V. S., Gallhofer, B., & Meyer-Lindenberg, A. (2005). Oxytocin modulates neural circuitry for social cognition and fear in humans. *Journal of Neuroscience*, 25, 11489–11493.

Kohrt, B. A., Hruschka, D. J., Kohrt, H. E., Carrion, V. G., Waldman, I. D., & Worthman, C. M. (2015). Child abuse, disruptive behavior disorders, depression, and salivary cortisol levels among institutionalized and community-residing boys in Mongolia. *Asia-Pacific Psychiatry*, 7, 7–19.

LeMoult, J., Ordaz, S. J., Kircanski, K., Singh, M. K., & Gotlib, I. H. (2015). Predicting first onset of depression in young girls: Interaction of diurnal cortisol and negative life events. *Journal of Abnormal Psychology*, 124, 850–859.

Levine, R. V., Reysen, S., & Ganz, E. (2008). The kindness of strangers revisited: A comparison of 24 US cities. *Social Indicators Research*, 85, 461–481.

Liu, R. X. (2016). School bonding, peer associations, and self-views: The influences of gender and grandparent attachment on adolescents in mainland China. *Youth and Society*, 48, 451–469.

Luke, N., Sinclair, I., Woolgar, M., & Sebba, J. (2014). *What works in preventing and treating poor mental health in looked after children?* London: NSPCC.

MacLean, P. D. (1990). *The triune brain in evolution: Role in paleocerebral functions.* Norwell, MA: Kluwer Academic Publishers.

MacMillan, H. L., Fleming, J. E., Streiner, D. L., Lin, E., Boyle, M. H., Jamieson, E., Duku, E. K., Walsh, C. A., Wong, M. Y.-Y., & Beardslee, W. R. (2001). Childhood abuse and lifetime psychopathology in a community sample. *American Journal of Psychiatry*, 158, 1878–1883.

Main, M., Kaplan, N., & Cassidy, J. (1985). Security in infancy, childhood, and adulthood: A move to the level of representation. *Monographs of the Society for Research in Child Development*, 50, 66–104.

McCrory, E., De Brito, S. A., & Viding, E. (2010). Research review: The neurobiology and genetics of maltreatment and adversity. *Journal of Child Psychology and Psychiatry*, 51, 1079–1095.

McCullough, E., Stedmon, J., & Dallos, R. (2014). Narrative responses as an aid to understanding the presentation of maltreated children who meet criteria for autistic spectrum disorder and reactive attachment disorder: A case series study. *Clinical Child Psychology and Psychiatry*, 19, 392–411.

Mehta, M. A., Golembo, N. I., Nosarti, C., Colvert, E., Mota, A., Williams, S. C. R., Rutter, M., & Sonuga-Barke, E. J. S. (2009). Amygdala, hippocampal and corpus callosum size following severe early institutional deprivation: The English and Romanian Adoptees study pilot. *Journal of Child Psychology and Psychiatry*, 50, 943–951.

Meins, E., Fernyhough, C., Arnott, B., Leekam, S. R., & Rosnay, M. (2013). Mind-mindedness and theory of mind: mediating roles of language and perspectival symbolic play. *Child Development*, 84, 1777–1790.

Meins, E., Fernyhough, C., de Rosnay, M., Arnott, B., Leekam, S. R., & Turner, M. (2012). Mind-mindedness as a multidimensional construct: Appropriate and nonattuned mind-related comments independently predict infant–mother attachment in a socially diverse sample. *Infancy*, 17, 393–415.

Meins, E., Fernyhough, C., Wainwright, R., Clark-Carter, D., Gupta, M. D., Fradley, E., & Tuckey, M. (2003). Pathways to understanding mind: Construct validity and predictive validity of maternal mind-mindedness. *Child Development*, 74, 1194–1211.

Meins, E., Fernyhough, C., Wainwright, R., Gupta, M. D., Fradley, E., & Tuckey, M. (2002). Maternal mind-mindedness and attachment security as predictors of theory of mind understanding. *Child Development*, 73, 1715–1726.

Midgley, N., & Vrouva., I. (Eds.). (2012). *Minding the child: Mentalization-based interventions with children, young people and their families.* London: Routledge.

Mills, R., Scott, J., Alati, R., O'Callaghan, M., Najman, J. M., & Strathearn, L. (2013). Child maltreatment and adolescent mental health problems in a large birth cohort. *Child Abuse & Neglect*, 37, 292–302.

Morhenn, V. B., Park, J. W., Piper, E., & Zak, P. J. (2008). Monetary sacrifice among strangers is mediated by endogenous oxytocin release after physical contact. *Evolution and Human Behavior*, 29, 375–383.

Morris, A. S., Silk, J. S., Steinberg, L., Myers, S. S., & Robinson, L. R. (2007). The role of the family context in the development of emotion regulation. *Social Development*, 16, 361–388.

Moule, R. K., Decker, S. H., & Pyrooz, D. C. (2013). Social capital, the life-course, and gangs. In C. L. Gibson & M. D. Krohn (Eds.), *Handbook of life-course criminology* (pp. 143–158). New York: Springer.

Muris, P., Mayer, B., & Meesters, C. (2000). Self-reported attachment style, anxiety, and depression in children. *Social Behavior and Personality. An International Journal*, 28, 157–162.

Music, G. (2010). *Nurturing natures: Attachment and children's emotional, social and brain development.* London: Psychology Press.

Ogden, P. (2006). *Trauma and the body: A sensorimotor approach to psychotherapy* (1st ed.). New York: W. W. Norton & Co.

Opacka-Juffry, J., & Mohiyeddini, C. (2011). Experience of stress in childhood negatively correlates with plasma oxytocin concentration in adult men. *Stress*, 15, 1–10.

Panksepp, J., & Biven, L. (2012). *The archaeology of mind: Neuroevolutionary origins of human emotion.* New York: Norton.

Porges, S. W. (2011). *The polyvagal theory: Neurophysiological foundations of emotions, attachment, communication, and self-regulation.* New York: Norton.

Posada, G., & Jacobs, A. (2001). Child–mother attachment relationships and culture. *American Psychologist*, 56, 821–822.

Pressman, S. D., Black, L. L., & Segerstrom, S. C. (2012). Positive emotions and immunity. In S. Sergestrom (Ed.), *The Oxford handbook of psychoneuroimmunology* (pp. 92–104). Oxford: Oxford University Press.

Price, L. H., Kao, H. T., Burgers, D. E., Carpenter, L. L., & Tyrka, A. R. (2012). Telomeres and early-life stress: An overview. *Biological Psychiatry*, 73, 15–23.

Prior, V., & Glaser, D. (2006). *Understanding attachment and attachment disorders: Theory, evidence and practice.* London: Jessica Kingsley.

Raby, K. L., Cicchetti, D., Carlson, E. A., Cutuli, J. J., Englund, M. M., & Egeland, B. (2012). Genetic and caregiving-based contributions to infant attachment: Unique associations with distress reactivity and attachment security. *Psychological Science*, 23, 1016–1023.

Robertson, J. (1971). Young children in brief separation – A fresh look. *Psychoanalytic Study of the Child*, 26, 264–315.

Rothbaum, F., & Morelli, G. F. (2005). Attachment and culture: Bridging relativism and universalism. In W. Friedlmeier, P. Chakkarath & B. G. Schwarz (Eds.), *Culture and human development: The importance of cross-cultural research for the social sciences* (pp. 99–124). London: Routledge.

Sagi, A., van IJzendoorn, M. H., Aviezer, O., Donnell, F., Koren-Karie, N., Joels, T., & Harel, Y. (1995). Attachments in a multiple-caregiver and multiple-infant environment: The case of the Israeli kibbutzim. *Monographs of the Society for Research in Child Development*, 60, 71–91.

Sameroff, A., Gutman, L. M., & Peck, S. C. (2003). Adaptation among youth facing multiple risks: Prospective research findings. In S. Luthar (Ed.), *Resilience and vulnerability: Adaptation in the context of childhood adversities* (pp. 364–391). New York: Cambridge University Press.

Sampson, N. R., Parker, E. A., Cheezum, R. R., Lewis, T. C., O'Toole, A., Patton, J., Zuniga, A., Robins, T. G., & Keirns, C. C. (2013). A life course perspective on stress and health among caregivers of children with asthma in Detroit. *Family and Community Health*, 36, 51–62.

Schoenmaker, C., Juffer, F., van IJzendoorn, M. H., Linting, M., van der Voort, A., & Bakermans-Kranenburg, M. J. (2015). From maternal sensitivity in infancy to adult attachment representations: A longitudinal adoption study with secure base scripts. *Attachment and Human Development*, 17, 241–256.

Schore, A. N. (1994). *Affect regulation and the origin of the self: The neurobiology of emotional development.* Mahwah, NJ: Lawrence Erlbaum.

Schwartz, J., & Begley, S. (2002). *The mind and the brain: Neuroplasticity and the power of mental force.* New York: Harper.

Sette, G., Coppola, G., & Cassibba, R. (2015). The transmission of attachment across generations: The state of art and new theoretical perspectives. *Scandinavian Journal of Psychology*, 56, 315–326.

Sigurdsson, T., Doyère, V., Cain, C. K., & LeDoux, J. E. (2007). Long-term potentiation in the amygdala: A cellular mechanism of fear learning and memory. *Neuropharmacology*, 52, 215–227.

Solms, M., & Panksepp, J. (2012). The 'Id' knows more than the 'Ego' admits: Neuropsychoanalytic and primal consciousness perspectives on the interface between affective and cognitive neuroscience. *Brain Sciences*, 2, 147–175.

Spangler, G. (2013). Individual dispositions as precursors of differences in attachment quality: why maternal sensitivity is nevertheless important. *Attachment and Human Development*, 15, 657–672.

Spence, S. H., O'Shea, G., & Donovan, C. L. (2015). Improvements in interpersonal functioning following interpersonal psychotherapy (IPT) with adolescents and their association with change in depression. *Behavioural and Cognitive Psychotherapy.* Online First, 1–16.

Sroufe, L. A. (2005). *The development of the person: The Minnesota study of risk and adaptation from birth to adulthood.* New York: Guilford Press.

Sroufe, L. A., & Waters, E. (1977). Attachment as an organizational construct. *Child Development*, 48, 1184–1199.

Stefini, A., Horn, H., Winkelmann, K., Geiser-Elze, A., Hartmann, M., & Kronmüller, K.-T. (2013). Attachment styles and outcome of psychoanalytic psychotherapy for children and adolescents. *Psychopathology*, 46, 192–200.

Stern, D. N. (1985). *The interpersonal world of the infant.* New York: Basic Books.

Strathearn, L. (2011). Maternal neglect: Oxytocin, dopamine and the neurobiology of attachment. *Journal of Neuroendocrinology*, 23, 1054–1065.

Strathearn, L., Iyengar, U., Fonagy, P., & Kim, S. (2012). Maternal oxytocin response during mother–infant interaction: Associations with adult temperament. *Hormones and Behavior*, 61, 429–435.

Tarren-Sweeney, M. (2010). It's time to re-think mental health services for children in care, and those adopted from care. *Clinical Child Psychology and Psychiatry*, 15, 613–626.

Tarren-Sweeney, M. (2013). An investigation of complex attachment- and trauma-related symptomatology among children in foster and kinship care. *Child Psychiatry and Human Development*, 44, 727–741.

Tarter, R. E., Kirisci, L., Gavaler, J. S., Reynolds, M., Kirillova, G., Clark, D. B., Wu, J., Moss, H. B., & Vanyukov, M. (2009). Prospective study of the association between abandoned dwellings and testosterone level on the development of behaviors leading to cannabis use disorder in boys. *Biological Psychiatry*, 65, 116–121.

Teicher, M. H., Dumont, N. L., Ito, Y., Vaituzis, C., Giedd, J. N., & Andersen, S. L. (2004). Childhood neglect is associated with reduced corpus callosum area. *Biological Psychiatry*, 56, 80–85.

Thomas, K. M., Drevets, W. C., Dahl, R. E., Ryan, N. D., Birmaher, B., Eccard, C. H., Axelson, D., Whalen, P. J., & Casey, B. J. (2001). Amygdala response to fearful faces in anxious and depressed children. *Archives of General Psychiatry*, 58, 1057–1063.

Thompson, E., & Cosmelli, D. (2011). Brain in a vat or body in a world?: Brainbound versus enactive views of experience. *Philosophical Topics*, 39, 163–180.

Tronick, E. (2007). *The neurobehavioral and social emotional development of infants and children.* New York: Norton.

True, M. M. M., Pisani, L., & Oumar, F. (2001). Infant–mother attachment among the Dogon of Mali. *Child Development*, 72, 1451–1466.

Van der Kolk, B. A. (2005). Developmental trauma disorder. *Psychiatric Annals*, 35, 401–408.

Van Niel, C., Pachter, L. M., Wade R. Jr, Felitti, V. J., & Stein, M. T. (2014). Adverse events in children: Predictors of adult physical and mental conditions. *Journal of Developmental and Behavioral Pediatrics*, 35, 549–551.

Weisman, O., Zagoory-Sharon, O., & Feldman, R. (2012). Oxytocin administration to parent enhances infant physiological and behavioral readiness for social engagement. *Biological Psychiatry*, 72, 982–989.

Wilkinson, R., & Pickett, K. (2009). *The spirit level: Why more equal societies almost always do better.* London: Allen Lane.

Yehuda, R., Engel, S. M., Brand, S. R., Seckl, J., Marcus, S. M., & Berkowitz, G. S. (2005). Transgenerational effects of posttraumatic stress disorder in babies of mothers exposed to the World Trade Center attacks during pregnancy. *Journal of Clinical Endocrinology and Metabolism*, 90, 4115–4118.

Zak, P. J. (2012). *The moral molecule: The new science of what makes us good or evil.* London: Bantam Press.

4

THERAPY OUTCOMES: IS CHILD THERAPY EFFECTIVE?

TERRY HANLEY AND JULIA NOBLE

This chapter discusses

- The impact of therapy upon the lives of children and young people
- The outcome of therapy for children and young people in real world settings
- The complexity of measuring change in therapeutic work with children and young people
- How children, young people, parents and teachers view therapy

Introduction

Within this chapter we provide an overview of the **research** examining the outcomes of therapy with children and young people. At the heart of this discussion we consider the concept of **evidence-based practice** and whether therapy is **effective** with this age group. Further, we also reflect upon some of the key issues that are encountered when measuring therapeutic outcomes. Before continuing however, and for those who might be impatient, the simple answer to this question appears to be 'yes, it is effective'. Analysis of outcome studies in this area does demonstrate that children and young people commonly benefit from therapeutic interventions. However, like most simple answers, there is more to this than meets the eye!

Box 4.1 Evidence-based practice

This is an approach to patient care that encourages the integration of research knowledge from clinical trials and outcome studies, with clinical judgement and patient values, to inform therapeutic work.

The efficacy of therapy for children and adolescents

Traditionally, it has been argued that there has been a focus on applying the findings of studies conducted with adults to work with young people (Hanley, Sefi, Cutts, & Pattison, 2013). As we understand more about the unique nature of the child/adolescent–therapist relationship, and how developmental milestones have their own psychological impact, this is no longer seen to be appropriate. As a consequence, there have now been at least 1,500 clinical trials examining therapeutic interventions with young people (Durlak, Wells, Cotten, & Johnson, 1995; Kazdin, 2000) spanning over five decades (Weisz, Ugueto, Cheron, & Herren, 2013). These clinical trials are commonly known as **randomized controlled trials** (RCTs) and are described in Box 4.2.

Box 4.2 What is a randomized controlled trial?

RCTs are commonly considered the 'gold standard' of research evidence. They are an experimental study in which participants are randomly assigned to two or more groups, such that the efficacy of the different interventions can be identified.

The results from clinical trials have been incorporated into **meta-analyses**, which combine the findings from a number of studies to try and establish an overall effect. These meta-analyses generally conclude that therapy proves beneficial for children and young people. For example,

- Casey and Berman (1985) found a mean **effect size** of 0.71 when looking at 75 outcome studies with children aged 12 and younger, and 0.79 for studies with 4–18 year olds.
- Weisz, Weiss, Alicke and Klotz (1987) report a mean effect size of 0.79 for 106 studies with 4–18 year olds.
- Kazdin, Bass, Ayers and Rodgers (1990) found a mean effect size of 0.88 for treatment versus no-treatment comparisons, and 0.77 for comparisons of treatment groups and active **control groups** when looking at 223 studies of 4–18 year olds.
- Weisz, Weiss, Han, Granger and Morton (1995) found a mean effect size of 0.71 when looking at 150 studies with individuals aged between 2 and 18.

Box 4.3   How do we do know if a young person or group of young people have improved or not?

Statistical significance

- When looking at the outcomes of therapy it is important for us to know whether the change in young people is as a result of attending therapy or whether any difference is just due to chance. Researchers do this by setting an acceptable level of risk that the change observed was due to chance, rather than due to the intervention (typically, 1 in 20, or 0.05). If the actual data suggest a probability that is less than this, we then say the results are **statistically significant** – the two groups (which could be before and after therapy, or one type of therapy against other) are different. If the probability value is calculated at more than 0.05 then this does not automatically mean the intervention was ineffective, it just means that it is more likely that the difference between the two groups is due to chance.

Critique of statistical significance

- Although the *p*-value is an extremely widely used approach it has limitations (Cohen, 1969). For instance, the threshold of 0.05 is completely arbitrary, and statistical significance is tied to sample size. This means larger samples are more likely to find a statistical difference whereas small samples are less likely to achieve statistical significance and therefore important differences that are genuinely present might be missed. For further discussion of this, see Gigerenzer (2004) and Goldacre (2014). An alternative and widely used approach to the concept of statistical significance is **effect size**.

Effect size

- In outcome research, effect sizes indicate the magnitude of difference between two groups. This is important because a group of young people might have significantly lower scores on a depression measure after eight weeks of counselling, but this does not tell us what this actually means in someone's life. Effect size is one statistical way of describing this. The most commonly used effect size in outcome research is Cohen's *d*. Cohen (1969) provided guidance on interpreting effect sizes, stating an effect size of 0.2 was small, 0.5 was medium and in terms of therapeutic change would amount to a noticeable improvement in symptoms, and 0.8 was large. However, when interpreting these figures caution is warranted as these values have been derived from more medical sciences. Therefore, there is an argument to say the effectiveness of an intervention can only be interpreted in relation to other similar interventions.

Clinically significant change

- Shifts in outcomes scores that are meaningful (for example, from scores that are typical for clinical populations to scores that are more typical of non-clinical populations) can be calculated in different ways, usually based on population norms for that measure (the most obvious is looking at patients who score over clinical cut-offs at one time point, but later on a score below the cut-off).

In summary, drawing this evidence together, therapy helps about 75 per cent of young clients (see Weisz, Sandler, Durlak, & Anton, 2005 for further discussion here). Such research provides compelling evidence and can prove very influential with policy makers. As with all research findings however, the positive view that therapy 'works' is not as straightforward as it may first seem.

Rather than considering whether therapy 'works' in a very broad sense, as with therapy for adults, the debate has moved on. Much research now focuses upon which therapeutic approaches have the best outcomes for which problems – what works for whom, and why? A detailed look at which approaches appear to work best for specific problems will not however be considered here as it is the focus of Chapter 5.

Box 4.4   Implications for practice

The findings from clinical trials indicate that counselling and psychotherapy are efficacious strategies for supporting children and young people who encounter difficulties in their lives.

Box 4.5   Efficacy, effectiveness and outcomes

Efficacy

Efficacy studies measure the potential for change under optimal conditions, or to put it another way at any cost (for example, regardless of **cost-effectiveness** or practicality). Most RCTs are efficacy studies: for example do 12 sessions of manualized cognitive behavioural therapy (CBT) improve young people's self-reported measures of depression? These findings are then considered alongside results from a comparison/control group.

Effectiveness

Effectiveness studies measure the potential for change in the real world (without the support associated with more controlled research). For example: do the 12 sessions of manualized CBT improve self-reported measures of depression in a child and adolescent mental health service? These findings can then be contrasted to a comparison group of people on a waiting list not receiving therapy.

Outcomes

Outcome studies may also look at the result of providing a therapeutic intervention, but without a comparison to a group not receiving the therapy. For example, what is the change in self-reported depression scores at the end of therapy with this young person or group of young people when compared to the scores at the outset of therapy?

Change in the real world: The outcomes of therapy

When considering therapeutic outcomes, why do we need to look at evidence from the real world? Is it not possible to use the findings from clinical trials and apply these to practice? Well, as Weisz and Gray (2008) point out, the evidence suggests that everyday clinical practice is characterized by interventions that do not rely on behavioural and cognitive principles, or clinical trial literature. In the sections that follow we therefore consider a number of important questions related to the findings of real world, practice-based evidence.

Box 4.6   Practice-based evidence

This is the systematic collection of information about particular therapeutic approaches or methods (namely the use of outcome measures) within real world settings.

Outcome data from the Child Outcomes Research Consortium (CORC) (see Box 4.7) have reported that there is commonly a reduction in symptoms and improvement in general wellbeing following a therapeutic intervention for young people. This is most notably evident in Wolpert et al.'s (2012) study of outcome measure data from over 16,000 individual encounters between young people and practitioners from 41 child and adolescent mental health services (CAMHS). The researchers collected data on **standardized** patient-reported outcomes, clinician-reported outcomes and **idiographic** goal-based outcomes with young people and their family members. Across all measures of outcome there was a **statistically significant** change, and modest but robust effect size change, which was greater than would be expected without any therapeutic intervention. These findings are generally consistent with previous studies, which have shown modest but significant improvements in mental health outcomes following therapy in practice-based settings (Ford, Hutchings, Bywater, Goodman, & Goodman, 2009).

The British Association for Counselling and Psychotherapy (BACP) conducted a large review of 138 therapeutic interventions and found evidence suggesting cognitive behavioural therapy, psychodynamic therapy, play therapy and humanistic therapies have all been shown to be effective with children and adolescents (McLaughlin, Holliday, Clarke, & Ilie, 2013). The review highlighted that more studies have researched the effects of cognitive behavioural therapy (36 per cent of total studies) than any other type of therapy and, as such, there is a need for research exploring the effects of other therapies. The BACP review also identified key factors that influenced the effectiveness of therapeutic approaches, across a range of problems. These were race, gender, ethnicity, the child–therapist alliance and parental involvement. Generally, matched gender, race and ethnicity and a strong therapeutic alliance between young person and therapist positively impacted on a young person's motivation and likelihood of staying in therapy. Parental involvement was also seen to be beneficial when working with younger children, particularly in play therapy.

The picture is not always positive, with older meta-analyses of usual clinical care being found to have effect sizes averaging about zero and thus indicating no benefit (for example, Weisz, 2004; Weisz, Donenberg, Han, & Weiss, 1995). It would appear that the picture has changed for the better; however further exploration of routine therapeutic work is clearly needed.

Box 4.7 Child Outcomes Research Consortium (CORC)

The Child Outcomes Research Consortium (www.corc.uk.net/) is a national not-for-profit organization in the UK which provides advice on recommended measures to use with young people. By encouraging the collection of **routine outcome measures** in services, CORC aims to evaluate service provision and improve understanding of young people's mental and well-being issues.

What outcomes do we use to measure change?

When attempting to measure whether therapy 'works' or not, we first need to understand what types of change(s) we are attempting to capture (e.g. progress in therapy, overall outcome, symptoms, or assessment for particular disorders). As such, a staggering number of measures have been developed for use in child and adolescent therapy. Johnston and Gowers (2005) systematically reviewed the research literature and identified 113 different measures. Given the vast array it can be difficult to know which one (or selection) to use with each client to strike a balance between the competing demands of reliability, validity and feasibility. A helpful review of 100 different measures used routinely by clinicians in CAMHS by Wolpert et al. (2008) is a good starting point to learn more about which specific measures to use in different circumstances (see recommended reading at the end of this chapter).

Who do we ask to measure change in young people?

A number of people might be involved in assessing the outcome of therapy with children and young people. For instance, parents or teachers might be asked to provide ratings of the strengths and difficulties that they may encounter, or expert raters might be involved in providing diagnoses. These external perspectives are sought because asking children and young people themselves to complete questionnaires to assess their subjective experiences is viewed as commonly more complex than with adults (depending on the age of the child). This can be more difficult due to their developmental capabilities: for example, how do we know they understand the question being asked? Therefore, it is really important when using an outcome measure with children and young people that it is valid (it was developed with children and young people in mind and has been tested on them in development). Most outcome measure questionnaires for children and young people will have been designed for a narrow age range as children and adolescents' brain development is phenomenal – what an individual at age 6 can understand is vastly different to age 10

(De Luca et al., 2003). This is very different to adults, where brain development is not dramatically different between the ages of 31 and 34 – or we hope not!

Do young people, parents and others agree on the outcome of therapy?

As mentioned earlier, there are many ways of measuring change in children and adolescents (for example, interviews and observations of young people). Many of these methods are similar to ways of measuring change in adults, however, with young people it is a lot more common to get multiple sources of information about the young person from parents, families, teachers and other significant people in their life. This enables us to **triangulate** (see Box 4.8) findings and build up a picture of the young person's life. However, we have to be cautious about this as multi-informant perspectives rarely straightforwardly agree. For example, Humphrey, Kalambouka, Wigelsworth, Lendrum, Lennie and Farrell (2010) evaluated the effects of a short intervention on mental health in primary schools using child self-report and parent and teacher perspectives. They reported significant change in the child report but no difference from the perspectives of parents and teachers. A similar finding was reported in adolescents by Duncan, Sparks, Miller, Bohanske and Claud (2006), who noted that adolescents rate themselves less distressed than caregivers do. This can be quite confusing, and brings up the question of which perspective is considered the most important for therapy to be deemed as effective.

Box 4.8   Triangulation

Triangulation involves bringing together multiple sources of information to form a more detailed picture based on what all these sources are pointing towards. It is a term often used in research when more than one method is used to collect data.

Do some young people get worse in therapy?

Very little information exists on the percentage of children and young people who get worse in therapy. Therapy with this age group throws up some unique challenges when considering why young people might not get better, however. DiGiuseppe, Linscott and Jilton (1996) point out that young people do not commonly self-refer and frequently come to therapy in a resistant, 'precontemplative' stage of change. French, Reardon and Smith (2003) go even further and suggest that some young people can be even forced into therapy. These inherent difficulties have led several researchers to suggest that some child and adolescent clients might not have sufficient understanding of therapy to make use of the 'space' provided (Shirk & Saiz, 1992).

Kazdin (2004) reports that 40–60 per cent of young people drop out of therapy. Although we cannot conclude from this that young people drop out because they were getting worse, as they might have dropped out as they were feeling better, it is still a concerning figure.

Box 4.9   Dropping out of therapy

There can be numerous reasons for individuals dropping out of therapy. An individual may feel that it is no longer needed because their therapeutic goals have been sufficiently addressed or that it is not meeting their needs. In the case of the latter, a poor therapeutic alliance might be one factor. Shirk, Karver and Brown (2011) state the alliance is an important predictor of youth therapy outcomes and may well be an essential ingredient that makes diverse child and adolescent therapies work (see further discussion of therapeutic alliance in Chapter 6).

The reason that individuals attend therapy might also be important. One study, exploring a service for 12–25 year olds, noted that individuals with internalized problems, relationship problems and who were older were less likely to drop out, while those with externalizing problems, homelessness and who were younger were more likely to drop out (Baruch, Vrouva, & Fearon, 2009).

How much therapy do clients need?

Due to the individual nature of a child or young person's difficulties we cannot say for sure how much therapy any individual will need. However, studies looking at the average length of sessions and/or the impact of session length have given us some indication of what currently exists and whether or not it works. For instance, the 2013 BACP review, cited above, states that the length of therapy when working with children and adolescents tends to be less than 12 sessions (although the review was largely influenced by CBT research), and that this tends to be effective (McLaughlin et al., 2013). This was supported by McArdle (2007), who critiqued a review of the evidence for depression in children and young people conducted by the National Institute for Health and Care Excellence (NICE) and firmly recommended psychological treatment should be offered for at least three (and potentially six) months. One study that examined the impact of short-term versus long-term psychodynamic therapy for young people (aged 6–18 years) concluded both approaches were effective; however a long-term approach was more effective (Kronmuller, Stefini, Geiser-Elze, Horn, Hartmann, & Winkelmann, 2010).

When considering the length of therapy, some of the difficulties inherent in adult therapy come into play. For instance, the need to balance children becoming overly dependent on the therapy or perceiving themselves as inherently defective, alongside trying to ensure long-lasting change. Some of the literature around play therapy warns against short-term therapy in children who have witnessed traumatic experiences, as the therapy might be perceived as another loss if it is withdrawn too quickly (Wilson & Ryan, 2005). However, a large body of evidence for short-term interventions has shown improvements in symptoms (McLaughlin et al., 2013). In short, there is not a clear answer to this question and more research is needed to see the impact of length of therapy on outcomes.

On a different note, Chu and Harrison (2007) found session length affected outcomes. They found longer sessions had a greater effect than short ones in young people aged 6–18 years showing symptoms of seasonal affective disorder, generalized anxiety disorder, depression or social phobia. Such a finding contrasts with some practices which reduce session length to fit with individual needs and would once again be a territory for further exploration.

Does the impact of therapy continue beyond the end of therapy?

Meta-analyses of therapeutic outcomes suggest the benefits of therapy with children and adolescents are maintained after therapy (when considered at five- to six-month follow-ups) (e.g. Weisz et al., 1987; Weisz, Weiss, et al., 1995). The research in this area is however still relatively limited. For instance, McLaughlin et al. (2013) highlight that some studies conduct six- or 12-month follow-up but rarely longer term.

The studies which have followed up young people in the short to medium term indicate the gains from therapy are maintained. This appears to be the case across different presenting problems, therapeutic approaches, cultures and children with learning disabilities (Feeny, Foa, Treadwell, & March, 2004; Gilboa-Schechtman et al., 2010; Rosenberg, Jankowski, Fortuna, Rosenberg, & Mueser, 2011; Schechtman & Pastor, 2005).

In one of the few studies which did measure long-term impact of therapy (12 sessions of CBT), Carpentier, Silovsky and Chaffin (2006) found improvement in symptoms was maintained 10 years later. Such a finding might indicate that therapy has a long-lasting impact. Moreover, some research has suggested that these effects can even be increased after therapy has ended. In a systematic review looking at the effects of psychodynamic psychotherapy over a broad geographical location, the authors concluded there was evidence of a 'sleeper' effect – which is to say symptomatic recovery was greater at six months follow-up than at the end of therapy (McLaughlin et al., 2013). However, clearly further investigation of such a phenomenon is needed prior to firm conclusions being drawn.

Is therapy better than other alternatives?

In a society that requires therapeutic services across the board to continually justify their worth, it is important to consider therapy alongside alternative forms of support. Below we consider the literature around the cost-effectiveness of therapy with young people alongside the two approaches that might be viewed as more economic in nature, notably whole school approaches and medication.

Is therapy cost-effective?

In the modern age, cost-effectiveness plays a big part of most funded services as limited resources mean that tough decisions have to made on where to allocate budgets. It is very difficult to calculate the cost associated with having a mental health problem and therefore whether therapy is a viable option or provides better value than alternatives. As Knapp (2003) points out, to calculate the full costs of mental ill health, it is necessary to include not just the healthcare and other service and capital costs but also the associated human costs, including the impact on carers. A school-based initiative in the UK, Place2Be estimated the total cost of having a mental health problem over childhood (9–15 years) is £32,346 (2007/8 prices), compared to the cost of providing therapy in a specialist CAMHS service which they estimated as £1,744 per individual per year or £954 for their one-to-one school-based counselling service (Place2Be, 2010).

All these costs are estimates and as there have been limited studies completed in this area we cannot form conclusions, but this initial research would indicate having some form of intervention is cost-effective. This perspective raises even more questions, such as which interventions are most effective taken into account their associated cost? Salloum (2010) suggests that in order to increase access to treatment for children, lower cost interventions, such as minimally assisted CBT or group approaches, might be a good option as part of a stepped care model. We will now consider some of these other interventions.

Whole school initiatives

Whole school approaches move beyond learning and teaching to introduce into schools a focus on emotional health and wellbeing. A number of different initiatives have been developed and evaluated, such as the Social and Emotional Aspects of Learning (SEAL) programme, which was designed to create an ethos and climate in schools to promote social and emotional skills. The evaluation had mixed results, finding 50 per cent of teachers perceived that pupil listening skills had improved and 44 per cent perceived pupil concentration levels had improved (Humphrey et al., 2008).

Other interventions have reported more positive outcomes, the Penn Resilience Program implemented an 18-lesson curriculum for 11–13 year olds to develop skills such as emotional intelligence, flexible and accurate thinking, self-efficacy, assertive communication and problem-solving. Three local authorities in England piloted the programme. The evaluation found the programme had a positive impact on pupils' application of skills to real life situations, a short-term improvement in depression symptom scores, school attendance rates and academic attainment in English, and an overall greater impact for the most vulnerable groups (Challen, Noden, West, & Machin, 2011).

Other similar programmes have also demonstrated whole school approaches benefit young people (Durlak, Weissberg, Dymnicki, Taylor, & Schellinger, 2011). As such we can say that school-level interventions have highlighted a potential cost-effective future design for supporting the mental health of children and adolescents. However, as Durlak and DuPre (2008) point out, there are barriers to overcome before these programmes can be rolled out as standard practice. For instance, the teachers' 'will and skill', conflicting priorities, access to resources and ability to provide these interventions within educational budgets all become relevant.

To date there has been very little consideration of how individual therapy and whole school initiatives work together, with reviews of the literature highlighting the challenge of multidisciplinary working (Cooper, Evans, & Pybis, 2016). Further, no comparisons of individual therapy and whole school initiatives have been conducted.

Medication

Medication is a controversial topic in the area of child and adolescent mental health and beyond the scope of this book. However, we will attempt to provide a very brief synopsis for you to start to consider this area. Most practitioners and parents would, we imagine, prefer that a young person is not on medication, considering we know that some medications cause long-term structural changes in the brain (Andersen, 2005). This is backed up by the views of young people themselves. In a survey of 156 adolescents

Bradley, McGrath, Brannen and Bagnell (2010) found a higher preference for psychotherapy than antidepressants.

The research evidence investigating the effects of medication compared to therapy is mixed. In the largest cited trial focusing upon young people with a diagnosis of depression, March, Silva and Vitiello (2006) compared CBT with fluoxetine (an antidepressant) and placebo. They found fluoxetine was superior to CBT, and CBT was equivalent to placebo. However, in a meta-analysis looking at the reduction in psychological harm in adolescents under 21 who had experienced traumatic experiences comparing different types of therapy and medication, Wethington et al. (2008) concluded CBT was effective but there was insufficient evidence to draw conclusions about the effect of medication. Why the conflicting findings? It could be that medication is helpful for some problems and some individuals and not for others. Kennard et al. (2009) found individuals who show no response to treatment with an antidepressant responded positively to a CBT intervention. In conclusion, we can say it looks like medication can have positive outcomes for some young people, but whether or not this is better than other approaches is uncertain.

Box 4.10   Implications for practice

Practitioners should be aware of the dynamics of working with other professionals and the potential impacts of other interventions that run parallel to work with children and young people (for example, school-based interventions and medication).

Box 4.11   Does monitoring our own practice improve outcomes?

- Why do we need to measure change in our work? As a clinician working closely with young people, don't we just know or sense when a young person is improving or not in therapy? Actually the answer to this is probably not. Research has shown that we are actually pretty inaccurate at measuring whether people have improved in therapy (Hannan et al., 2005). Therefore to get an answer to whether therapy works for young people we need ways of measuring it. Using standardized measures embedded within therapy can be one way of monitoring outcomes. With this in mind, the BACP recommend a selection of questionnaires that can be used for working with children and young people (McLaughlin et al., 2013). Two of these are: The Child Outcome Rating Scale (CORS) (Duncan et al., 2006) for under 13 years and the Outcome Rating Scale (ORS) for 13 years and over (Miller, Duncan, Brown, Sparks, & Claud, 2003) provide a brief measure of global distress suitable for assessing treatment outcome. It a very brief four-item measure which takes only a few minutes to complete and score.
- The Young Person's Clinical Outcomes in Routine Evaluation (YP-CORE) was developed by Twigg, Barkham, Bewick, Mulhern, Connell and Cooper (2009) and measures psychological distress in 11–16 year olds. It consists of 10 items and has risk and clinical cut-off scores to aid interpretation.

How do young people, parents and teachers view therapy?

Qualitative research can provide a rich understanding of the processes that go on within therapy. As such it can help ensure that the perspectives of young people and others associated with them are taken into account when evaluating therapy. Approaches such as interviews and focus groups can aid our understanding of how an intervention has (or has not) worked as well as raising important issues such as helpful and unhelpful factors. This can be essential in helping develop relevant ways of working with this client group; as Castro-Blanco and Karver (2010) point out, the intervention might be the best in the world, but it is effectively useless if there is no one there to receive it. Below we provide an overview of some salient qualitative research in this area.

Box 4.12   Qualitative research

This is research based on language and does not use numbers or statistics.

How do children and young people view therapy?

There has been relatively little research exploring how children and young people view therapy. The relative neglect of children's views appears, in part, to stem from uncertainty about the capacity of children to express their views reliably (Meadows, 2012). In the past few decades researchers have questioned this view and it is now established practice to place a high significance on the child's perspective (Day, Carey, & Surgenor, 2006). Research has also established the child's perspective is different from a caregiver or teacher, and therefore we cannot approximate their views from an adult close to them (Stith, Rosen, McCollum, Coleman, & Herman, 1996; Strickland-Clark, Campbell, & Dallos, 2000).

Several researchers (Everall & Paulson, 2002; Gibson & Cartwright, 2013; Lynass, Pykhtina, & Cooper, 2012) have acknowledged that consulting and listening to young people is essential for the future development of effective services. Griffiths' (2013) review of the helpful and unhelpful factors that young people report in school-based counselling proved no different and provides a useful summary of the literature in this area. It identified nine relevant studies, with the most frequently reported factor being the opportunity to talk to someone and be listened to. Other factors included an opportunity to get things off their chest, to feel understood, accepted and not judged. The quality of the relationship was not the only component reported to be helpful by young people. They also discussed the need for counsellors to use strategies and provide guidance. These included:

- problem-solving activities
- guidance by way of advice and suggestions
- teaching insight to develop more awareness of self and others
- asking questions
- strategies for dealing with problems
- demonstrating particular techniques such as relaxation exercises.

Young people have also reported that the context in which therapy is offered proves to be an important factor. Pattison, Rowland, Richards, Cromarty, Jenkins and Polat (2009) found young people highlighted the importance of therapy being:

- embedded within their daily routine, to help avoid any associated stigma and disruption;
- confidential, so as to create a safe space;
- neutral, and not being with a known other such as a family member or teacher.

Some of these requirements raise potential challenges as therapy with young people often means information is shared between the therapist and relevant parties such as parents, teachers and social services.

Young people have also talked about specific factors which impact on their motivation to participate in therapy (Day et al., 2006). These were convenient appointment times and that, for these individuals, activities proved preferable to talking. They also highlighted therapists asking questions can cause discomfort. This is demonstrated in the quotes below:

> You don't know them and they want you to tell them what's going on in your life and you don't really know them and you're not that much confident . . . they should get to know you first and you get to know them and then they can ask. (Child 5) (p. 148)

> There's too much questions . . . couldn't keep up and it was frightening cos . . . didn't know what was happening. (Child 4) (p. 149)

Such views contrast, however, to other research which notes that some individuals like being asked questions as it gives therapy a direction (for example, Cooper, 2009; Griffiths, 2013). Ultimately, such opposing comments reflect the varied wants and needs that young clients present with.

What is it helpful for?

Lynass et al. (2012) interviewed young people who expressed predominantly positive views of school-based counselling with changes in three main domains, emotional, interpersonal and behavioural. Participants viewed these changes as having had an important effect on their lives. This has been supported by numerous sources which report that promoting mental health in children and young people has a positive impact on learning, achievement, attendance and behaviour (Department for Education and Skills, 2001; Pattison & Harris, 2006; Pettit, 2003). It is not known exactly how this occurs, although Durlak (1997) suggests a potential ripple effect where counselling and psychotherapy enhances social and emotional attainment and this increases academic, behavioural and mental health aspects.

How do parents/families view therapy?

Relatively few studies have explored the views of parents and families towards therapy, focusing mainly on parental levels of satisfaction with services (Bradley & Clark, 1993;

Byalin, 1993; Heflinger, Sonnichsen, & Brannan, 1996). In one of the few studies in this area, Hilton, Turner, Krebs, Volz and Heyman (2012) looked at parental satisfaction with child mental health assessment at a specialist service for young people with a diagnosis of obsessive-compulsive disorder. The researchers found during assessment that parents value being told about their child's strengths as well as their difficulties and appreciate having time to explain their concerns and an opportunity to speak to clinicians without their child present in the room.

Stallard (1995) assessed parental satisfaction with a child and adolescent psychology service using a postal questionnaire and follow-up interviews. Out of 57 families, 75 per cent were satisfied overall with the service, 61 per cent said the situation had changed for the better following contact with the service, and 77 per cent said the service had helped them to deal with their problems. One study looked at the comparison between parents (or caregivers) and young people's opinion of services through self-report questionnaires (Barber, Tischler, & Healy, 2006). The researchers found high levels of satisfaction for both groups, although the children and adolescents were less satisfied than the parents/carers. There was little or no agreement between parents/carers and children/adolescents on most questions. The only question in which young people and parents/carers were in agreement was 'How easy is it to get here?', which would be expected as we would imagine they would travel together! This demonstrates just how different the needs and views of young people might be compared to their families.

How do teachers view therapy?

In Cooper's (2009) review of school-based counselling the views of teachers' responses to therapy were collated. On average, just over 80 per cent of teachers who responded rated counselling as moderately or very helpful, with teachers giving it a mean rating of 8.22 on a 10-point scale of helpfulness. Such positive findings have also been echoed in evaluations of counselling in schools in Wales (Hill et al., 2011) and England and Scotland (Hanley, Jenkins, Barlow, Humphrey, & Wigglesworth, 2012).

Qualitative responses (through open-ended questionnaire items and/or interviews) from teachers were also brought together in Cooper's (2009) review. These indicated why they thought counselling was helpful or unhelpful to pupils. Five factors identified as helpful were:

- the neutrality of the therapist, meaning someone other than teachers or parents that a young person could talk to;
- confidentiality, which referred to the private nature of the therapy service;
- accessibility, meaning that young people could be referred to the therapy service easily, and without long delays;
- expertise, meaning the therapist's specialized training;
- time, teachers noting that the counsellor, in contrast to themselves, can spend extended amounts of time with a young person.

Other factors teaching staff cited as helpful were that therapy was non-stigmatizing and non-directive. The unhelpful factors cited by school staff in two or more studies were that they wanted:

- greater availability, hoping that the counselling service could be extended, with more counsellors and/or for more hours per week;
- greater promotion of the service within school;
- more therapeutic activities than just one-to-one counselling to be offered (such as anger management groups and counselling for parents);
- better communication, with counsellors being more open with staff (such as providing more feedback on how clients are doing);
- more advice giving.

In the above, it is easy to see here how there can be conflicts between the needs of young people and the requirements of others (for example, teachers): while young people expressed a need for privacy, teachers requested more transparency, for instance. Further, it highlights how difficult it can be to meet the needs of all stakeholders while still maintaining the therapeutic relationship with the young person.

Box 4.13   Implications for practice

The qualitative research highlights the need for practitioners to proactively listen to the views of key stakeholders in the therapeutic process. These 'experts through experience' provide important insights into the helpful and unhelpful aspects of the work we do.

Summary of key findings

- There is a large amount of evidence to suggest that psychological therapies have a positive effect on children and adolescents' mental health and wellbeing.
- Meta-analyses of experimental designed research suggest that 75 per cent of children and young people who attend therapy benefit from it.
- Contemporary practice-based evidence generally reflects the positive impact that therapy has upon young people's lives.
- There are over 100 different measures for considering outcomes (these reflect upon progress in therapy, overall outcomes, specific symptoms and assess particular disorders).
- Some research suggests that between 40 and 60 per cent of children and young people drop out of therapy.
- Therapy for children and adolescents is commonly short-term (below 12 sessions). At present there is little research to confirm whether length of therapy is linked to outcome.
- Young people are generally positive about their experiences of therapy. They commonly report having someone to talk to (and be listened to) as the most helpful component of therapy.
- Parents, families and teachers generally find therapeutic services helpful and report being satisfied with what they offer.

Recommended reading

McLaughlin, C., Holliday, C., Clarke, B., & Ilie, S. (2013). *Research on counselling and psychotherapy with children and young people: A systematic scoping review of the evidence for its effectiveness from 2003–2011.* Lutterworth: British Association for Counselling and Psychotherapy. This paper was commissioned by the BACP to review the evidence for counselling and young people and gives an excellent overview of the research in this area.

MindEd (www.minded.org.uk) provides a number of e-learning resources for working with children and young people. This includes information on utilizing process and outcome measures within practice.

Wolpert, M., Aitken, J., Syrad, H., Munroe, M., Saddington, C., Trustam, E., et al. (2008). *Review and recommendations for national policy for England for the use of mental health outcome measures with children and young people.* London: Report for Department for Children, Schools and Families and Department of Health. This is a comprehensive review of outcome measures used in children and young people research.

Questions for reflection

- Do you think making therapeutic decisions based on research evidence always leads to the best outcomes with children and young people? If so, why? If not, why not?
- If we have multiple perspectives (child, parent and teacher) on whether therapeutic change has occurred, whose perspective is most important? And what are the implications of this?
- Consider your own views on outcome measures. How might these impact upon your work with young people? Are there any other things to bear in mind when trying to judge whether a therapy is helping a child or adolescent client?

References

Andersen, S. L. (2005). Stimulants and the developing brain. *Trends in Pharmacological Sciences,* 26, 237–243.

Barber, A. J., Tischler, V. A., & Healy, E. (2006). Consumer satisfaction and child behaviour problems in child and adolescent mental health services. *Journal of Child Health Care,* 10, 9–21.

Baruch, G., Vrouva, I., & Fearon, P. (2009). A follow-up study of characteristics of young people that drop out and continue psychotherapy: Service implications for a clinic in the community. *Child and Adolescent Mental Health,* 14, 69–75.

Bradley, E., & Clark, B. (1993). Patients' characteristics and consumer satisfaction on an inpatient child psychiatric unit. *Canadian Journal of Psychiatry/ Revue Canadienne de psychiatrie,* 38, 175–180.

Bradley, K. L., McGrath, P. J., Brannen, C. L., & Bagnell, A. L. (2010). Adolescents' attitudes and opinions about depression treatment. *Community Mental Health Journal,* 46, 242–251.

Byalin, K. (1993). Assessing parental satisfaction with children's mental health services: A pilot study. *Evaluation and Program Planning,* 16, 69–72.

Carpentier, M. Y., Silovsky, J. F., & Chaffin, M. (2006). Randomized trial of treatment for children with sexual behavior problems: Ten-year follow-up. *Journal of Consulting and Clinical Psychology,* 74, 482–488.

Casey, R. J., & Berman, J. S. (1985). The outcome of psychotherapy with children. *Psychological Bulletin*, 98, 388–400.

Castro-Blanco, D. E., & Karver, M. S. (Eds.). (2010). *Elusive alliance: Treatment engagement strategies with high-risk adolescents*. Washington, DC: American Psychological Association.

Challen, A., Noden, P., West, A., & Machin, S. (2011). UK resilience programme evaluation: Final report. Department for Education.

Chu, B. C., & Harrison, T. L. (2007). Disorder-specific effects of CBT for anxious and depressed youth: A meta-analysis of candidate mediators of change. *Clinical Child and Family Psychology Review*, 10, 352–372.

Cohen, J. (1969). *Statistical power analysis for the behavioral sciences*. New York: Academic Press.

Cooper, M. (2009). Counselling in UK secondary schools: A comprehensive review of audit and evaluation data. *Counselling and Psychotherapy Research*, 9, 137–150.

Cooper, M., Evans, Y., & Pybis, J. (2016). Interagency collaboration in children and young people's mental health: A systematic review of outcomes, facilitating factors and inhibiting factors. *Child: Care, Health and Development*, 42, 325–342.

Day, C., Carey, M., & Surgenor, T. (2006). Children's key concerns: Piloting a qualitative approach to understanding their experience of mental health care. *Clinical Child Psychology and Psychiatry*, 11, 139–155.

De Luca, C. R., Wood, S. J., Anderson, V., Buchanan, J.-A., Proffitt, T. M., Mahony, K., & Pantelis, C. (2003). Normative data from the CANTAB. I: Development of executive function over the lifespan. *Journal of Clinical and Experimental Neuropsychology*, 25, 242–254.

Department for Education and Skills. (2001). *Promoting children's mental health in the early years and in school settings*. London: DfEE Publications.

DiGiuseppe, R., Linscott, J., & Jilton, R. (1996) Developing the therapeutic alliance in child–adolescent psychotherapy. *Applied and Preventive Psychology*, 5, 85–100.

Duncan, B., Sparks, J., Miller, S. D., Bohanske, R., & Claud, D. (2006). Giving youth a voice: A preliminary study of the reliability and validity of a brief outcome measure for children, adolescents, and caretakers. *Journal of Brief Therapy*, 5, 66–82.

Durlak, J. A. (1997). Current status and future directions. *Successful prevention programs for children and adolescents* (pp. 177–201). New York: Springer.

Durlak, J. A., & DuPre, E. P. (2008). Implementation matters: A review of research on the influence of implementation on program outcomes and the factors affecting implementation. *American Journal of Community Psychology*, 41, 327–350.

Durlak, J. A., Weissberg, R. P., Dymnicki, A. B., Taylor, R. D., & Schellinger, K. B. (2011). The impact of enhancing students' social and emotional learning: A meta-analysis of school-based universal interventions. *Child Development*, 82, 405–432.

Durlak, J. A., Wells, A. M., Cotten, J. K., & Johnson, S. (1995). Analysis of selected methodological issues in child psychotherapy research. *Journal of Clinical Child Psychology*, 24, 141–148.

Everall, R. D., & Paulson, B. L. (2002). The therapeutic alliance: Adolescent perspectives. *Counselling and Psychotherapy Research*, 2, 78–87.

Feeny, N. C., Foa, E. B., Treadwell, K. R., & March, J. (2004). Posttraumatic stress disorder in youth: A critical review of the cognitive and behavioral treatment outcome literature. *Professional Psychology: Research and Practice*, 35, 466–476.

Ford, T. J., Hutchings, J., Bywater, T., Goodman, A., & Goodman, R. (2009). Evaluation of the Strengths and Difficulties Questionnaire Added Value Score as a method for estimating effectiveness in child mental health interventions. *The British Journal of Psychiatry*, 194, 552–557.

French, R., Reardon, M., & Smith, P. (2003). Engaging with a mental health service: Perspectives of at-risk youth. *Child and Adolescent Social Work Journal*, 20, 529–548.

Gibson, K., & Cartwright, C. (2013). Agency in young clients' narratives of counseling: 'It's whatever you want to make of it'. *Journal of Counseling Psychology*, 60, 340–352.

Gigerenzer, G. (2004). Mindless statistics. *The Journal of Socio-Economics*, 33, 587–606.

Gilboa-Schechtman, E., Foa, E. B., Shafran, N., Aderka, I. M., Powers, M. B., Rachamim, L., et al. (2010). Prolonged exposure versus dynamic therapy for adolescent PTSD: A pilot randomized controlled trial. *Journal of the American Academy of Child and Adolescent Psychiatry*, 49, 1034–1042.

Goldacre, B. (2014). *Bad pharma: How drug companies mislead doctors and harm patients*. Basingstoke: Macmillan.

Griffiths, G. (2013). *Helpful and unhelpful factors in school-based counselling: Clients' perspectives*. Lutterworth: British Association for Counselling and Psychotherapy.

Hanley, T., Jenkins, P., Barlow, A., Humphrey, N., & Wigglesworth, M. (2012). *A scoping review of the access to secondary school counselling*. Manchester: University of Manchester.

Hanley, T., Sefi, A., Cutts, L., & Pattison, S. (2013). Research into youth counselling: A rationale for research informed pluralistic practice. In T. Hanley, N. Humphrey & C. Lennie (Eds.), *Adolescent counselling psychology: Theory, research and practice* (pp. 88–108). London: Routledge.

Hannan, C., Lambert, M. J., Harmon, C., Nielsen, S. L., Smart, D. W., Shimokawa, K., & Sutton, S. W. (2005). A lab test and algorithms for identifying clients at risk for treatment failure. *Journal of Clinical Psychology*, 61, 155–163.

Heflinger, C. A., Sonnichsen, S. E., & Brannan, A. M. (1996). Parent satisfaction with children's mental health services in a children's mental health managed care demonstration. *The Journal of Mental Health Administration*, 23, 69–79.

Hill, A., Cooper, M., Pybis, J., Cromarty, K., Pattison, S., Spong, S., Dowd, C., Leahy, C., Counchman, A., Rogers, J., Smith, K., & Maybanks, N. (2011). *Evaluation of the Welsh school-based counselling strategy: Final report*. Cardiff: Welsh Government Social Research.

Hilton, K., Turner, C., Krebs, G., Volz, C., & Heyman, I. (2012). Parent experiences of attending a specialist clinic for assessment of their child's obsessive compulsive disorder. *Child and Adolescent Mental Health*, 17, 31–36.

Humphrey, N., Kalambouka, A., Bolton, J., Lendrum, A., Wigelsworth, M., Lennie, C., & Farrell, P. (2008). *Primary social and emotional aspects of learning (SEAL): Evaluation of small group work*. London: Department for Children, Schools and Families.

Humphrey, N., Kalambouka, A., Wigelsworth, M., Lendrum, A., Lennie, C., & Farrell, P. (2010). New beginnings: Evaluation of a short social-emotional intervention for primary-aged children. *Educational Psychology*, 30, 513–532.

Johnston, C., & Gowers, S. (2005). Routine outcome measurement: A survey of UK child and adolescent mental health services. *Child and Adolescent Mental Health*, 10, 133–139.

Kazdin, A. (2000). *Psychotherapy for children and adolescents: Directions for research and practice*. Oxford: Oxford University Press.

Kazdin, A. E. (2004). Psychotherapy for children and adolescents. In M. J. Lambert (Ed.), *Bergin and Garfield's handbook of psychotherapy and behavior change* (pp. 543–589). New York: Wiley.

Kazdin, A. E., Bass, D., Ayers, W. A., & Rodgers, A. (1990). Empirical and clinical focus of child and adolescent psychotherapy research. *Journal of Consulting and Clinical Psychology*, 58, 729–740.

Kennard, B. D., Clarke, G. N., Weersing, V. R., Asarnow, J. R., Shamseddeen, W., Porta, G., et al. (2009). Effective components of TORDIA cognitive-behavioral therapy for adolescent depression: Preliminary findings. *Journal of Consulting and Clinical Psychology*, 77, 1033–1041.

Knapp, M. (2003). Hidden costs of mental illness. Editorial. *British Journal of Psychiatry*, 183, 477–478.

Kronmuller, K., Stefini, A., Geiser-Elze, A., Horn, H., Hartmann, M., & Winkelmann, K. (2010). The Heidelberg study of psychodynamic psychotherapy for children and adolescents. In J. Tsiantis & J. Trowell (Eds.), *Assessing change in psychoanalytic psychotherapy of children and adolescents* (pp. 115–138). London: Karnac.

Lynass, R., Pykhtina, O., & Cooper, M. (2012). A thematic analysis of young people's experience of counselling in five secondary schools in the UK. *Counselling and Psychotherapy Research*, 12, 53–62.

March, J., Silva, S., & Vitiello, B. (2006). The Treatment for Adolescents with Depression Study (TADS): Methods and message at 12 weeks. *Journal of the American Academy of Child and Adolescent Psychiatry*, 45, 1393–1403.

McArdle, P. (2007). Comments on NICE guidelines for 'depression in children and young people'. *Child and Adolescent Mental Health*, 12, 66–69.

McLaughlin, C., Holliday, C., Clarke, B., & Ilie, S. (2013). *Research on counselling and psychotherapy with children and young people: A systematic scoping review of the evidence for its effectiveness from 2003–2011*. Lutterworth: British Association of Counselling and Psychotherapy.

Meadows, S. (2012). *The child as thinker: The development and acquisition of cognition in childhood*. London and New York: Routledge.

Miller, S. D., Duncan, B., Brown, J., Sparks, J., & Claud, D. (2003). The outcome rating scale: A preliminary study of the reliability, validity, and feasibility of a brief visual analog measure. *Journal of Brief Therapy*, 2, 91–100.

Pattison, S., & Harris, B. (2006). Counselling children and young people: A review of the evidence for its effectiveness. *Counselling and Psychotherapy Research*, 6(4), 233–237.

Pattison, S., Rowland, N., Richards, K., Cromarty, K., Jenkins, P., & Polat, F. (2009). School counselling in Wales: Recommendations for good practice. *Counselling and Psychotherapy Research*, 9, 169–173.

Pettit, B. (2003). Effective joint working between CAMHS and schools: DfES Research Report RR412.

Place2Be. (2010). Positive outcomes for children and families: An economic analysis of The Place2Be's integrated school-based services for children.

Rosenberg, H. J., Jankowski, M. K., Fortuna, L. R., Rosenberg, S. D., & Mueser, K. T. (2011). A pilot study of a cognitive restructuring program for treating posttraumatic disorders in adolescents. *Psychological Trauma: Theory, Research, Practice, and Policy*, 3, 94–99.

Salloum, A. (2010). Minimal therapist-assisted cognitive-behavioral therapy interventions in stepped care for childhood anxiety. *Professional Psychology: Research and Practice*, 41, 41–47.

Shechtman, Z., & Pastor, R. (2005). Cognitive-behavioral and humanistic group treatment for children with learning disabilities: A comparison of outcomes and process. *Journal of Counseling Psychology*, 52, 322–336.

Shirk, S. R., & Saiz, C. C. (1992). Clinical, empirical, and developmental perspectives on the therapeutic relationship in child psychotherapy. *Development and Psychopathology*, 4, 713–728.

Shirk, S. R., Karver, M. S., & Brown, R. (2011). The alliance in child and adolescent psychotherapy. *Psychotherapy*, 48, 17–24.

Stallard, P. (1995). Parental satisfaction with intervention: Differences between respondents and non-respondents to a postal questionnaire. *British Journal of Clinical Psychology*, 34, 397–405.

Stith, S. M., Rosen, K. H., McCollum, E. E., Coleman, J. U., & Herman, S. A. (1996). The voices of children: Preadolescent children's experiences in family therapy. *Journal of Marital and Family Therapy*, 22, 69–86.

Strickland-Clark, L., Campbell, D., & Dallos, R. (2000). Children's and adolescent's views on family therapy. *Journal of Family Therapy*, 22, 324–341.

Twigg, E., Barkham, M., Bewick, B. M., Mulhern, B., Connell, J., & Cooper, M. (2009). The Young Person's CORE: Development of a brief outcome measure for young people. *Counselling and Psychotherapy Research*, 9, 160–168.

Weisz, J. R. (2004). *Psychotherapy for children and adolescents: Evidence-based treatments and case examples*. Cambridge: Cambridge University Press.

Weisz, J. R., & Gray, J. S. (2008). Evidence-based psychotherapy for children and adolescents: Data from the present and a model for the future. *Child and Adolescent Mental Health*, 13, 54–65.

Weisz, J. R., Donenberg, G. R., Han, S. S., & Weiss, B. (1995). Bridging the gap between lab and clinic in child and adolescent psychotherapy. *Journal of Consulting and Clinical Psychology*, 63, 688–701.

Weisz, J. R., Sandler, I. N., Durlak, J. A., & Anton, B. S. (2005). Promoting and protecting youth mental health through evidence-based prevention and treatment. *American Psychologist*, 60, 628–648.

Weisz, J. R., Ugueto, A. M., Cheron, D. M., & Herren, J. (2013). Evidence-based youth psychotherapy in the mental health ecosystem. *Journal of Clinical Child and Adolescent Psychology*, 42, 274–286.

Weisz, J. R., Weiss, B., Alicke, M. D., & Klotz, M. L. (1987). Effectiveness of psychotherapy with children and adolescents: A meta-analysis for clinicians. *Journal of Consulting and Clinical Psychology*, 55, 542–549.

Weisz, J. R., Weiss, B., Han, S. S., Granger, D. A., & Morton, T. (1995). Effects of psychotherapy with children and adolescents revisited: A meta-analysis of treatment outcome studies. *Psychological Bulletin*, 117, 450–468.

Wethington, H. R., Hahn, R. A., Fuqua-Whitley, D. S., Sipe, T. A., Crosby, A. E., Johnson, R. L., et al. (2008). The effectiveness of interventions to reduce psychological harm from traumatic events among children and adolescents: A systematic review. *American Journal of Preventive Medicine*, 35, 287–313.

Wilson, K., & Ryan, V. (2005). *Play therapy: A non-directive approach for children and adolescents*. London: Elsevier Health Sciences.

Wolpert, M., Aitken, J., Syrad, H., Munroe, M., Saddington, C., Trustam, E., et al. (2008). *Review and recommendations for national policy for England for the use of mental health outcome measures with children and young people*. London: Report for Department for Children, Schools and Families and Department of Health.

Wolpert, M., Ford, T., Trustam E., Law, D., Deighton, J., Flannery, H., & Fugard, R. J. (2012). Patient-reported outcomes in child and adolescent mental health services (CAMHS): Use of idiographic and standardized measures. *Journal of Mental Health*, 21, 165–173.

5

THERAPY OUTCOMES: WHAT WORKS FOR WHOM?

PETER FONAGY, LIZ ALLISON AND ALANA RYAN

This chapter discusses

- What we mean by evidence-based practice
- The evidence base for the treatment of different kinds of childhood problems with different forms of psychological therapy
- The limits of our knowledge about what works for whom
- The implications of the evidence base for clinical practice and research

Introduction

While the evidence base for what works for whom remains limited, there is an increasing body of research that clinicians can draw on to inform their practice with children and young people. In order to make the best use of the information that is available, it is important both to be familiar with the existing evidence and to be aware of its limitations.

What do we mean by evidence-based practice?

We need to begin with a caveat. Evidence-based practice (EBP) cannot be assured by 'choosing' a treatment from a list of approved options. Historically, there has been a tendency to assume that a treatment can be 'branded' once and for all as an EBP so that no further reflection on how, or for whom, to implement it is needed. It is extremely important to avoid idealizing evidence in this way. While the existence of evidence increases the chances of a treatment being effective, it does not guarantee success. Reviews of the **empirical** literature aim to identify what works, but systematic study of the literature actually reveals that many of the people who receive evidence-based treatments experience no change. It is very important that our statements about the **effectiveness** (or ineffectiveness) of particular approaches in this chapter are read with this caveat in mind. Research on the features of practising evidence-based care in mental health has identified that in addition to being consistently science-informed, it is organized around client intentions, culturally sensitive (it considers the context in which the clinician is practising relative to the context in which the evidence was originally gathered), and continually monitors the effectiveness of interventions, adapting as necessary to serve the client better (APA Presidential Task Force on Evidence-Based Practice, 2006; Spring, 2007). This chapter focuses on the first item in this set of components, but it should not be forgotten that the latter require an active stance on the clinician's part (Sackett, Rosenberg, Gray, Haynes, & Richardson, 1996). For example, the endpoint for a given treatment will be more appropriately determined by ongoing assessment of outcome for a particular child than by the average length of treatment derived from a number of **randomized controlled trials** (RCTs; see Box 5.8) (Daleiden & Chorpita, 2005).

How can child and adolescent counsellors and therapists use this chapter?

While it may not be necessary to read through this whole chapter, when thinking about setting up a service, or when a new referral comes in, the practitioner may want to look at the relevant section of this chapter before considering treatment recommendations. The findings reported here should then of course be considered alongside other factors informing the practitioner's judgement, such as client preference.

Overview of the evidence for the treatment of childhood problems with psychological therapies

Below we briefly review the evidence for the use of psychological therapies to treat a range of diagnosable childhood disorders. We also consider evidence for the psychological treatment of the difficulties associated with experiences of maltreatment.

Box 5.1 Defining mental health problems in childhood

This chapter is organized according to DSM-IV (American Psychiatric Association, 1994) rather than DSM-5 categories (American Psychiatric Association, 2013) because the research literature we are considering has mostly used the former. However, there is current controversy about the validity of DSM diagnostic categories which cannot easily be dismissed (see, for example, Cuthbert & Insel, 2013). Specifically, many within the research community have acknowledged that using the **outcomes** data from short-term, highly controlled interventions with somewhat arbitrarily defined client groups to inform the design of the services provided for a set of long-term, quite heterogeneous conditions, is problematic. Similarly, others have challenged the hegemony of medical diagnoses, noting that adherence to strict diagnostic criteria is not the only way we can define a problem. In any setting, we encounter a child, not a diagnosis, and they may not fall neatly into a particular diagnostic category. These issues have also led to the emergence of alternative definitional approaches such as the National Institute of Mental Health's Research Domain Criteria (RDoC) project, which aims to develop a more integrative research classification system for mental disorders. This system is based on dimensions of neurobiology – which considers how the nervous system influences cognitive and behavioural patterns – and observable behaviour that cuts across the current diagnostic categories.

Anxiety disorders

Generalized anxiety disorder (GAD)	A form of anxiety which can be triggered by many different things and which can occur on a daily basis. It can be longer-lasting than other anxiety subtypes.
Social anxiety disorder (SAD)/Social phobia (SP)	A form of anxiety prompted by a persistent and intense fear of day-to-day social situations. It can result in the person being unable to participate in social events or peer group activities.
Obsessive-compulsive disorder (OCD)	A form of anxiety disorder which is characterized by the presence of inescapable unpleasant thoughts and urges which are temporarily relieved by the repetition of certain routines or processes.
Post-traumatic stress disorder (PTSD)	An anxiety disorder which manifests following a particularly stressful or alarming experience. Symptoms can include continuous re-experience of traumatic memory, insomnia, irritability and unwillingness to address and process the traumatic memory.

Cognitive behavioural therapy (CBT)

Meta-analyses offer strong support for CBT as a good place to start when considering how to treat anxiety (Cartwright-Hatton, Roberts, Chitsabesan, Fothergill, & Harrington, 2004; In-Albon & Schneider, 2007; Ishikawa, Okajima, Matsuoka, & Sakano, 2007; James, Soler, & Weatherall, 2005), although it should be noted that RCTs in which CBT was compared with a credible alternative treatment are relatively scarce.

Box 5.2 Why meta-analysis?

In a given study, the size of the sample has a substantial impact on the likelihood of finding a **statistically significant difference** between treatment and **control** conditions. Meta-analyses pool multiple studies and summarize outcomes by plotting and aggregating the differences between the means obtained in treatment and control conditions. This method substantially increases the reliability of the estimate of the likely size of treatment effects even when the studies on which it is based are relatively small. For this reason, in this chapter we often consider available meta-analyses before turning to individual studies. However, it should be kept in mind that if there is a limited evidence base or significant heterogeneity among studies, meta-analytic estimates should be treated cautiously.

Children and young people with generalized anxiety disorder (GAD), social anxiety disorder (SAD) or social phobia (SP) who are treated with certain CBT packages, such as Coping Cat, Coping Koala and FRIENDS, improve more than those on a waiting list for the same treatment (Kendall, 1994; Kendall, Hudson, Gosch, Flannery-Schroeder, & Suveg, 2008; Lau, Chan, Li, & Au, 2010; Silverman, Kurtines, Ginsburg, Weems, Lumpkin, & Carmichael, 1999). These programmes aim to help children and young people recognize anxiety warning signs, while also teaching relaxation and resilience strategies. Coping Cat has two main parts: skills training and skills practice, and involves one-to-one work with a therapist. Coping Koala and FRIENDS are programmes which bring many children together to work with a therapist in a group setting. By working as part of a team, Coping Koala and FRIENDS enable children to share common experiences and develop ways to beat anxiety collectively. In fact, research shows that about 50–60 per cent of those treated with these programmes are likely to recover. Studies of Coping Cat have shown that its effects last for up to a year, and possibly even longer (Kendall, Safford, Flannery-Schroeder, & Webb, 2004; Kendall et al., 2008). However, this kind of treatment for anxiety does not seem to reduce the risk of developing a mood disorder (anxiety or depression) later in life. We do not know very much about how CBT performs when compared with an attention placebo, that is, an alternative control treatment which is akin to CBT in terms of time and effort, but which has no therapeutic value or **treatment as usual** (TAU), namely the care routinely offered for the person's condition in a community clinic. The few studies that have been done so far suggest that its effects may be much smaller than when it is compared with a **wait-list control** (Barrington, Prior, Richardson, & Allen, 2005; Southam-Gerow, Weisz, Chu, McLeod, Gordis, & Connor-Smith, 2011). When CBT treatment takes place in a community clinic, it may not be significantly more effective than usual treatment, but there are not enough studies to be sure about this, and usual treatment probably includes many of the effective components of CBT.

Group CBT appears to be as effective as individual CBT and is cheaper (Liber et al., 2008; Manassis et al., 2002). Individual CBT may possibly be better at improving depression and other internalizing disorder symptoms (i.e. non-verbalized negative mood patterns which can also manifest as withdrawal, somatic problems and anxiety) (Saavedra, Silverman, Morgan-Lopez, & Kurtines, 2010), but more studies are needed to confirm whether this is the case. While we do not know whether involving families in individual and group CBT leads to better or worse outcomes, or makes no difference, there is evidence to suggest that when parents themselves are very anxious, involving them in the child's treatment can be helpful

(Cobham, Dadds, & Spence, 1998). Indeed, recent analysis suggests that for children aged nine or younger, training the parents in CBT methods may be just as effective as child-focused CBT (Waters, Ford, Wharton, & Cobham, 2009).

CBT can be made more accessible in various ways, including bibliotherapy and computerized CBT (cCBT), sometimes enhanced with telephone or email contact. While the first method encourages the young person to explore specific texts which may boost resilience to anxiety, the second approach uses short online courses to help children and young people and their families learn specific coping techniques. Neither treatment necessitates seeing a therapist, yet treatment effects have been maintained for up to a year (Spence et al., 2011). We need to know more about how cCBT compares to clinic-based CBT for young people with anxiety. One study has suggested that it is just as effective (Spence et al., 2011), although only about a third of the young people recovered. Clearly, more research is needed. Giving teachers, nurses, parents and the affected children themselves a role in delivering treatment also increases its accessibility (e.g. Galla et al., 2012).

However, CBT may not work for everyone with an anxiety disorder. The existing evidence suggests that it may be less effective with more severely affected and less well-supported children (e.g. Southam-Gerow, Kendall, & Weersing, 2001). Its effectiveness also depends on the quality of the service, and it is unlikely to work if delivered by clinicians who have not received adequate training.

The effects of CBT for obsessive-compulsive disorder (OCD) have been shown to last for as long as six to nine months after the end of treatment (e.g. Piacentini et al., 2011). Less input from the therapist may be needed when the treatment includes use of client workbooks (Bolton et al., 2011). CBT is less likely to work for children and young people with a family history of OCD, unless they also receive antidepressant medication, such as selective serotonin reuptake inhibitors (SSRIs) (Garcia et al., 2010). We do not yet know for sure how large an impact we can expect CBT to have on OCD in children and young people. It appears possible that as few as 12 sessions of CBT can have a modest impact on OCD, and that daily sessions over a short period may be as effective as weekly sessions over several weeks (Storch, Lehmkuhl, Ricketts, Geffken, Marien, & Murphy, 2010), but more studies are needed to confirm these suggestions. It may be possible to deliver CBT for OCD effectively in ordinary clinical settings (Williams, Salkovskis, Forrester, Turner, White, & Allsopp, 2010), although its effects may be somewhat reduced; but again more research is required to substantiate this.

Trauma-focused CBT (TF-CBT), which uses cognitive and behavioural techniques to help children overcome traumatic experiences, is an effective treatment for post-traumatic stress disorder (PTSD) (Cary & McMillen, 2012), especially in treating trauma in sexually abused children and young people.

Several other therapies that use different components of TF-CBT also seem to be more effective than no treatment, including short-term cognitive processing therapy, which aims to help those who have experienced a trauma understand how this experience has affected their day-to-day lives, while also providing practical advice on how to manage their emotions (Ahrens & Rexford, 2002). The feasibility of treating children as young as three with TF-CBT has been explored (Scheeringa, Weems, Cohen, Amaya-Jackson, & Guthrie, 2011), but there is not enough evidence yet to be confident that this is a reasonable approach.

School-based CBT programmes for children and young people exposed to violence, such as the Cognitive Behavioral Intervention for Trauma in Schools (CBITS), have been shown to produce small but significant effects (Kataoka et al., 2003; Stein et al., 2003). CBITS can be administered either by clinically trained professionals or by school personnel without clinical training. It may be that while school-based treatments such as CBITS are more accessible than TF-CBT, they are somewhat less effective; but more research is needed to determine whether this is the case.

We do not know whether or not narrative exposure therapy (NET), which is based on the narrative exposure component of TF-CBT, is effective. The studies conducted so far have produced conflicting results (Ertl, Pfeiffer, Schauer, Elbert, & Neuner, 2011; Schaal, Elbert, & Neuner, 2009).

Other behavioural therapies

Simple phobias, such as an irrational fear of school, can be treated effectively by in vivo exposure (Roth & Fonagy, 2005), that is, receiving a gradual introduction to that which is feared. However, educational support may be just as effective (Silverman et al., 1999). School refusal can also be effectively treated by exposure (Last, Hansen, & Franco, 1998). Social effectiveness therapy (SET), a behavioural therapy programme which combines exposure with social skills training, is an effective treatment for social phobia (e.g. Beidel, Turner, & Young, 2006), and one study suggested that it was significantly more effective than SSRI treatment (with fluoxetine) (Beidel, Turner, Sallee, Ammerman, Crosby & Pathak, 2007). It is possible that SET may be slightly more effective than CBT for social phobia, but this hypothesis needs to be tested.

Exposure and response prevention (ERP) supported by cognitive interventions is an effective treatment for OCD. ERP works by breaking the association between the young person's obsessive thoughts and the subsequent behavioural compulsions which arise due to their stress or anxiety (Lewin, Storch, Geffken, Goodman, & Murphy, 2006).

We do not know whether eye movement desensitization and reprocessing (EMDR) for trauma symptoms in children and young people is effective (Field & Cottrell, 2011).

Psychodynamic psychotherapy

When psychodynamic psychotherapy is offered to parent and child (i.e. to families) rather than individual children, it can be effective (Lieberman, Van Horn, & Ghosh Ippen, 2005), especially where maltreatment or family trauma is involved (Ghosh Ippen, Harris, Van Horn, & Lieberman, 2011). Individual psychodynamic psychotherapy may be helpful for younger children with anxiety disorders (Muratori, Picchi, Bruni, Patarnello, & Romagnoli, 2003). Apart from these exceptions, we do not know whether or not psychodynamic therapies for children and young people with anxiety disorders are effective.

Box 5.3   Difficulties with evaluating psychodynamic psychotherapy

Psychodynamic psychotherapy is quite widely used, especially to treat children with entrenched and complex problems who have not responded to treatments for which there is a stronger evidence base, yet there have been few attempts to evaluate its effectiveness systematically (as is also the case with humanistic therapy and counselling), and the available studies often do not meet the methodological standards applied to the evaluation of much briefer and more goal-directed therapies. This is partly because of the complexities of designing such studies and partly because of their much greater costs. Until recently, child psychotherapies have rarely been manualized, and therefore grouping studies according to clinical method has not been possible. Studies of psychodynamic therapy have also tended to be less rigorous in identifying the diagnostic categories they address, or else have decided that it is not a fit with the model to design their research in relation to psychiatric diagnoses. Almost all studies of 'internalizing' children and young people consider a mixed group of anxious children with SAD, GAD, SP and OCD, with a limited number whose primary diagnosis may have been depression. In our subsequent discussions of treatments for specific diagnoses readers will note that often there is no mention of psychodynamic or humanistic approaches; this is because of the lack of available good quality evidence on whether or not they are effective for the problems we discuss.

Depression

Cognitive behavioural therapy

Whether it is provided individually or in a group setting, CBT appears to be an effective treatment for depression in young people (Munoz-Solomando, Kendall, & Whittington, 2008; Weisz, Jensen-Doss, & Hawley, 2006), although brief CBT does not reduce the chance of experiencing a subsequent episode (Birmaher et al., 2000). While many people suffering from depression do benefit from CBT, we do know that it is less likely to be of assistance to some. For instance, it is less effective where there are high levels of family conflict (Birmaher et al., 2000), where there is a history of sexual abuse (Barbe, Bridge, Birmaher, Kolko, & Brent 2004), or where cases are particularly complex, for example, where an adolescent is showing symptoms of emerging personality disorder (Birmaher et al., 2000). However, differences between CBT and other active treatments tend to disappear in longer-term follow-up studies (Birmaher et al., 2000). We do not know whether booster sessions of CBT improve outcomes, as different studies have reached different conclusions about this (Clarke, Rohde, Lewinsohn, Hops, & Seeley, 1999; Kroll, Harrington, Jayson, Fraser, & Gowers, 1996).

There is strong evidence for two particular CBT programmes: a highly structured, group-based intervention for depressed pre-adolescent girls (9–13 years) called ACTION (Stark, Hargrave, Hersh, Greenberg, Herren, & Fisher, 2008), and the Coping with Depression (CWDA) course for older teenagers (Clarke, Lewinsohn, & Hops, 1990). Both programmes are also effective with sub-threshold cases of depressive disorder (Beardslee et al., 2013; De Cuyper, Timbremont, Braet, De Backer, & Wullaert, 2004). Another version of CBT, the Pittsburgh programme, has been found to be more beneficial in the short-term than family therapy or more general therapy (Brent et al., 1997); the research undertaken to evaluate the Pittsburgh programme also found CBT to be less effective for individuals with a history of sexual abuse (Barbe et al., 2004) but more effective for those experiencing suicidal thinking (Birmaher et al., 2000).

It is unclear whether or not the Manchester programme of CBT for depression – a CBT manual which emphasizes explicit, tangible and shared goals, developed through clear structured sessions – is effective. Although the initial results of the programme were promising, especially for younger or less severely affected children and young people, a larger trial found that it brought no extra benefit when used in addition to the use of the SSRI fluoxetine (Goodyer et al., 2008).

Adopting a CBT approach to patient case management, i.e. ensuring that support for individuals with depression in community settings draws on some of the principles of this form of therapy, has been shown to improve outcomes in primary care (e.g. Lusk & Melnyk, 2011). Furthermore, applying CBT principles may also reduce the risk of depression. cCBT packages seem to produce comparable results to face-to-face counselling in the short-term at least (Merry, Stasiak, Shepherd, Frampton, Fleming, & Lucassen, 2012), but more studies are needed to confirm this.

Interpersonal psychotherapy

There is some evidence that therapy that is orientated towards the child or young person's relationships and their effect on mood; for example, interpersonal psychotherapy for adolescents (IPT-A), may be effective. However, when IPT-A is compared to other psychological treatments rather than attention placebo or minimal treatment, the results are not exceptional – it comes out as roughly as effective or slightly less effective (Rosselló & Bernal, 1999; Rosselló, Bernal, & Rivera-Medina, 2008). IPT-A may be better than CBT for more severe depression in some contexts (Gunlicks-Stoessel, Mufson, Jekal, & Turner, 2010), but more studies are needed to confirm this.

Family therapy

Family therapy is more effective than non-directive supportive therapy, but seems less effective than CBT (Brent et al., 1997). Attachment-based family therapy (ABFT), a form of therapy which focuses on intra-familial relationships with the aim of fostering a secure filial bond, may be particularly helpful with young people with severe levels of suicidal thinking (Diamond et al., 2010) – a group that has been observed to do poorly in conventional counselling. Multifamily psychoeducational approaches – structured programmes which provide families with information about specific disorders and skills training regarding how best to cope with them – may be more effective than doing nothing (Fristad, Verducci, Walters, & Young, 2009).

Psychodynamic psychotherapy

Psychodynamic psychotherapy may be better than doing nothing for young people with depression (Muratori et al., 2003) and may be as effective as systemic family therapy (Trowell et al., 2007), but more research is needed to confirm these suggestions. An adaptation of parent–child interaction therapy (PCIT), which draws on attachment theory in order to foster a safe and supportive relationship between parent and child, may be beneficial for pre-adolescent depression, but, again, further research is needed to confirm this (Lenze, Pautsch, & Luby, 2011).

Although we know that these different psychological therapies can, to varying degrees, have positive effects on childhood depression, a recent Cochrane review has concluded that there is still not enough evidence to say whether psychological therapies, antidepressants or a combination of the two is most effective for treatment of the disorder (Cox et al., 2014).

Non-directive supportive therapy

Following a systematic review of the literature, the NICE Guideline for the treatment of depression in children and young people recommended non-directive supportive therapy, which would include person-centred or humanistic approaches, as part of its stepped care model, recommending it for the treatment of mild depression without significant comorbid problems or signs of suicidal thoughts, if it still persists after a period of watchful waiting (National Institute for Health and Clinical Excellence, 2005). This recommendation was based on studies (Brent et al., 1997; Vostanis, Feehan, Grattan, & Bickerton, 1996) in which non-directive supportive interventions were used as comparators in studies of family therapy and CBT. Children and young people in these groups were found to benefit, and this recommendation still stands in the updated recommendations issued in 2015.

Conduct disorder

Oppositional defiant disorder (ODD)	Oppositional defiant disorder is characterized by a persistent pattern of defiance, anger and irritability when the child is confronted with authoritative figures, such as parents or teachers.
Conduct disorder (CD)	Unlike ODD, conduct disorder entails violation of others' basic rights or of age-appropriate social norms or rules. CD may be diagnosed on the basis of aggressiveness to people and animals, property destruction, deceptiveness or theft and/or serious rule violations.

Treatment for children under 11

Parent training

Given that social and familial environments can have a profound effect on the development or continuity of many mental health issues, therapy for parents which highlights how best to respond to their child's difficulties can be very beneficial. This is particularly true for conduct disorder (CD), for which parent training has been found to have a positive impact on children's behaviour (Drugli, Larsson, Fossum, & Morch, 2010). Training can be applied to a wide range of conduct problems and delivered effectively in various settings. However, it does not work for everyone, and while families at greatest risk often do respond to parent training, a substantial subgroup of families are not suited to this type of treatment and are likely to drop out (Fernandez & Eyberg, 2009; Hutchings, Bywater, Williams, Whitaker, Lane, & Shakespeare, 2011).

Parent training may be more effective if the child does not have other mental health difficulties, when the conduct problems are less severe, when the family has fewer socio-economic disadvantages, and when the parents are together and parental conflict and stress is low (Lundahl, Risser, & Lovejoy, 2006; Reyno & McGrath, 2006). Similarly, if the parents have high levels of social support and no history of antisocial behaviour or psychiatric difficulties themselves, a better outcome may be observed. More research is needed to confirm all these suggestions, however. It is unclear whether the effectiveness of parent training can be enhanced by adjunctive treatments, i.e. additional psychological or pharmacological treatment, for higher risk families, as different studies have reached different conclusions about this (Lundahl et al., 2006; National Institute for Health and Clinical Excellence, 2009).

It is also possible for parents to learn the necessary skills themselves, using a method known as self-directed parent training; however, it is unclear whether this is as effective as therapist-led parent training. Supportive evidence primarily stems from studies of parent training as a preventive measure, and requires confirmation in studies using clinical samples (Lundahl et al., 2006). This is especially important as there is also research showing that fidelity to **treatment protocol** and a high level of therapist skill are important in ensuring the success of parent training (Scott et al., 2010; Webster-Stratton & Reid, 2010).

Specific programmes for which there is evidence of effectiveness are discussed in Box 5.4.

Box 5.4 Parent training

Parent training is a behavioural family intervention conducted mainly with the child's parents, with limited therapist–child contact. Parents are encouraged to focus on prosocial behaviours rather than on the elimination of conduct problems. Treatment packages for which there is an evidence base include:

- The Incredible Years Program: a videotape modelling group discussion programme using a standard package of videotapes aimed at parents. The therapist leads a discussion of the interactions shown in short (two-minute) scenes on the videotapes and suggests structured homework exercises, including teaching play and reinforcement skills, effective limit-setting and non-violent discipline techniques, as well as problem-solving approaches.
- Triple P – Positive Parenting Program: an intensive parent training programme for parents of children with severe behavioural difficulties or who are at risk of developing such problems. Combines three delivery formats: group (eight sessions for groups of 10–12 parents, with telephone follow-up sessions), individual (10 sessions) and self-directed (a 10-week self-help programme augmented by telephone consultations).
- Oregon Social Learning Center (OSLC) Program: links the emergence of antisocial behaviour to coercive patterns of family interaction. Combines group treatment and individual family treatment. Homework is supported with midweek telephone calls aimed at promoting collaborative contact. Aims to replace coercive interactions with positive practices in five dimensions: (1) skill encouragement (scaffolding), (2) limit-setting, (3) monitoring of activities, whereabouts, peer contacts, etc., (4) problem-solving and (5) positive involvement (showing love and interest).
- PCIT: a two-phase therapy programme designed to teach parents to build a warm and responsive relationship with their child and to teach the child to behave appropriately. In the first phase (child-directed interaction), parents learn non-directive play skills

similar to those used by traditional play therapists. The aim is to change the quality of the parent–child relationship. In the second phase (parent-directed interaction), the parent learns, within the play interaction, to direct the child's play with clear, age-appropriate instructions. The emphasis is on consistent consequences, praise for compliance, and time-out for non-compliance.

While parent training can be a very powerful tool that works across cultures and different ethnic communities, it requires considerable involvement from the families concerned, and this can make it harder to get parents either to take up the treatment or to continue with it. For particularly 'hard-to-reach' or disadvantaged families, delivering parent training on a flexible, one-to-one basis rather than in a group setting produces better results (Lundahl et al., 2006). Improving positive parenting rather than reducing harsh or negative parenting is the most important factor in improving problem behaviour.

We do not know enough about how improvements in CD are maintained in the long-term following parent training. It seems that the programmes requiring the greatest input and commitment from both therapist and client/family are most likely to result in a long-term improvement, but we do not have enough evidence on whether intervening with parent training programmes might make the child less likely to become involved in criminal activity or substance use in adolescence (Lochman, Wells, & Lenhart, 2008; Lochman & Wells, 2003). More long-term follow-up studies are needed on all children with CD.

We also need more evidence as to whether it might be more effective to combine parent training with CBT for the child than to use either approach on its own, particularly in the case of children who have not benefited from parent training (Lochman, Boxmeyer, Powell, Barry, & Pardini, 2010; National Institute for Health and Clinical Excellence, 2009).

Box 5.5 Defining evidence-based treatments: General or specific?

Labels such as 'parent training' or 'CBT', attached in the mind of a reader to the conclusions of a study, will no more describe the content of the intervention than the label 'holiday' is likely to predict a family's experience of a specific summer vacation. There is a rapidly developing science of adherence measurement, which enables us to assess how closely treatment delivered in a particular context matches the protocol as originally designed. But in order to maintain the integrity of the combination of techniques that a particular EBP entails, there is a tendency to over-specify approaches, which can become a barrier to implementation. This is associated with a potential disadvantage for manualized therapies. When dealing with broad/heterogeneous groups of children exposed to multiple risk factors, such as poverty, poor parental mental health or negative peer influence, as well as children who suffer from multiple, co-occurring mental health disorders (comorbidities), the inflexibility of treatment manuals may prevent clinicians from recognizing and addressing specific issues that exist alongside the core presenting symptom that led to the children's inclusion in the trial. Treatment as usual, on the other hand, does have that flexibility, and can often be quite good. This makes it harder to demonstrate effectiveness of new interventions.

Cognitive behavioural therapy

CBT appears to be less effective than parent training as a treatment for conduct disorders in children (Bennett & Gibbons, 2000), although one meta-analysis suggested that when CBT was conducted in a clinical setting, the superiority of parent training over CBT was less pronounced (McCart, Priester, Davies, & Azen, 2006).

Cognitive behavioural methods that are designed to increase a child's self-control (i.e. anger management, social skills training) are moderately effective, although we know this mostly from studies of one particular intensive treatment package, the Coping Power Program, which requires its counsellors to undergo intensive training and needs a parenting component to achieve long-term effects on substance abuse and delinquency (Lochman & Wells, 2004).

Another child-oriented intervention – problem-solving skills training with parent management training, which combines elements of the Oregon Social Learning Center Program with cognitive approaches – improves the child's behaviour as well as improving family relations and reducing familial stress and parent dysfunction (Kazdin, 2010). These improvements are maintained at one-year follow-up. This intervention is less likely to be effective if the child is suffering from another mental health problem, belongs to an ethnic minority, has lower socio-economic status and/or has impaired cognitive and academic skills (Kazdin, 1997; Kazdin & Wassell, 2000; Kazdin & Whitley, 2006). It is more likely to work if the alliances between therapist, child and parent(s) are good.

Psychodynamic psychotherapy

There are no studies to show that psychodynamic treatments are effective for children with conduct problems. In the few studies available, the rates of improvement for psychodynamic therapy are lower than for other treatments, while the number of sessions needed is higher (Midgley & Kennedy, 2011).

School-based interventions

School-based interventions designed to change how teachers behave will not produce clinically significant improvements in individual children in the absence of other concurrent interventions. While classroom contingency management is helpful in controlling the behaviour of children while in that setting, it does not have a wider effect outside the classroom (Walker, Colvin, & Ramsey, 1995). If parents provide reinforcement by using similar strategies at home, e.g. to manage homework, the effectiveness of classroom-based support for behavioural problems may be enhanced (Forgatch & Ramsey, 1994; Kahle & Kelley, 1994).

School-wide anti-bullying interventions, which may include parent training, improved playground supervision, disciplinary methods, school conferences, videos, information for parents, classroom rules and classroom management, can reduce the amount of bullying that takes place in school (Farrington & Ttofi, 2009). We do not know how effective school-wide anti-bullying interventions are at reducing conduct problems or how many children participating in these interventions have oppositional defiant disorders or conduct disorder diagnoses.

Given that children with conduct problems often have distorted understandings of their social environment, it is possible that social learning theory-based interventions which modify and expand the child's interpersonal appraisal processes may be effective, but more research is needed to confirm this (National Institute for Health and Clinical Excellence, 2013).

Treatment for young people

Family-based approaches

Multimodal treatments combining different components (e.g. individual, family and/or group work) and involving the different systems that form the context for the adolescent's behaviour (family, school, peers, etc.) and which also have a family focus are the most likely to produce benefits that are maintained in the long-term, if they are well implemented (National Institute for Health and Clinical Excellence, 2013). The most effective of these treatments are intense, well-defined, yet capable of responding flexibly to unexpected situations, and deliver a range of interventions via the same therapist. However, even the most effective of these leave at least half of the young people treated with significant clinical problems.

In terms of specific family-based approaches, we know that multisystemic therapy (MST) is effective, and multidimensional family therapy (MDFT) also has an impact on CD (Liddle, Dakof, Turner, Henderson, & Greenbaum, 2008; Liddle, Dakof, Henderson, & Rowe 2011; Office of Program Policy Analysis and Government Accountability, 2007). Both are integrative and comprehensive family-based approaches which can be applied across many different contexts. Aligned to this, a similar 12–17 week programme of brief strategic family therapy, which focuses on the problem behaviours of the child as well as entire family functioning, can reduce behavioural problems (Santisteban et al., 2003). It is unclear whether brief strategic family therapy has a direct impact on delinquency. We do not know for sure whether multidimensional treatment foster care (MTFC) (an approach heavily influenced by the Oregon model, which involves placement with a specially trained foster family along with a package of other treatments) or functional family therapy (FFT, a phased, manualized and time-limited family therapy that aims to achieve changes in patterns of interaction and communication) are effective treatments for CD. Some studies have found benefits whereas others have failed to confirm this, and failures of replication may be associated with inadequate implementation of these interventions (Biehal, Ellison, & Sinclair, 2011; Sexton & Turner, 2010; Waldron, Slesnick, Brody, Turner, & Peterson, 2001; Westermark, Hansson, & Olsson, 2011). Thus far, behavioural parent training based on the Oregon model appears ineffective for young people and can be harmful when combined with group-based treatment for the adolescent (Dishion & Andrews, 1995).

Box 5.6   MST and MDFT

Multisystemic therapy (MST)

This is an ecological intervention that aims to impact on the entire milieu in which the young person operates. Constituent treatments include techniques from systemic and structural

(Continued)

(Continued)

family therapy, parent training, marital therapy, supportive therapy related to interpersonal problems, social skills components, social perspective training, behavioural methods and cognitive therapy techniques. as well as case management with the therapist acting as an advocate to outside agencies. Interventions are individualized and flexible but documented in treatment manuals. A family focus is key to the intervention.

Originally developed to treat conduct disorder, MST has also been used to treat self-injurious behaviour, substance use disorder, maltreated children and their parents.

Multidimensional family therapy (MDFT)

MDFT combines a highly structured manualized therapy with a flexible treatment delivery system titrated to the needs of the youth and family. It addresses multiple domains systematically: (a) within the adolescent, (b) within parents and other family members, (c) in the interactions between these individuals and (d) in extrafamilial systems (peers, education, etc.). Therapy consists of three phases: (a) establishing a foundation, (b) facilitating change and (c) consolidating change and 'launching' the adolescent.

Originally developed to treat substance use disorder in adolescents, MDFT has been used to treat conduct disorder.

Cognitive behavioural and social learning approaches

When cognitive behavioural and social learning approaches to CD in young people are tailored to the individual's specific needs and abilities and properly implemented, they are moderately effective, although change is less evident when these individuals are followed up. CBT may help to prevent adolescents in residential settings from reoffending. Social and problem-solving skills programmes and anger management training can produce improvements in social functioning and aggression (Sukhodolsky, Kassinove, & Gorman, 2004), but these improvements are only seen in the setting in which training takes place. Training in moral reasoning does not seem to have much of an impact on adolescent behaviour (Landenberger & Lipsey, 2005; Lipsey, Landenberger, & Wilson, 2007).

We do not know which of the many multicomponent CBT packages currently available delivers the greatest improvements, as this has not been systematically studied. The **efficacy** of alternative versions is likely to be influenced by what element or aspect of the package is most dominant. In fact, innovative reformulations of traditional CBT which place greater emphasis on personal acceptance and the therapeutic relationship, for example dialectical behaviour therapy (DBT) and mindfulness-based cognitive therapy, may have a positive impact on CD (Biegel, Brown, Shapiro, & Schubert, 2009; Drake & Barnoski, 2006), but more studies are needed to confirm this.

School-based interventions

Individual and group school-based treatments that target selected young people moderately reduce aggressive and disruptive behaviour regardless of differences in approach.

The Family Check-Up Program is an effective school-based treatment program targeting selected high-risk young people and their families (Dishion & Kavanagh, 2003). However, it must be noted that in the school setting, comprehensive treatment programmes are less effective than better targeted approaches (Wilson & Lipsey, 2007). The first tests of new school-based treatments usually produce the best results; when attempts are made to reproduce their effects on a larger scale these interventions have had partial success at best.

Integration with juvenile justice provision

Psychosocial treatments can be effectively integrated with juvenile justice provision, and when programmes divert juveniles from court processing this can reduce the likelihood of reoffending, especially when they are linked up with therapeutic services. In the United States, state-wide implementations of evidence-based community programmes have reduced crime and residential placements, although not all such implementations work equally well (Petrosino, Turpin-Petrosino, & Guckenburg, 2010). Residential programmes for antisocial youth which remove children from their social and familial networks for a set duration can make them worse rather than better. Wilderness programmes, which aim to tackle behavioural problems by supporting self-management and boosting resilience through outdoor adventure programmes, have a small positive impact on rates of reoffending and may improve family functioning (Bandoroff & Scherer, 1994; Harper & Russell, 2008). Wraparound services that seek to 'wrap' individualized services and support around the young person, rather than imposing a predetermined programme on them, seem to improve young people's living situations, but otherwise their impact on CD is small (Suter & Bruns, 2008, 2009).

High-quality implementation (carrying out the treatment in a way that is consistent with the treatment developers' original intention) seems to be as important as the type of intervention in producing good outcomes, since 'generic' psychosocial treatments such as mentoring and group counselling can be effective if they are implemented well and aimed at high-risk offenders. Multicomponent interventions (which offer different types of therapy in various combinations, but are not integrated by an overarching focus or set of principles) are ineffective (National Institute for Health and Clinical Excellence, 2009).

Surprisingly, older teenagers and those at higher risk of offending are slightly more likely to benefit from treatment (Andrews & Bonta, 2006; Lipsey, 2009). Treatments have the smallest impact on sexual offenders (Redondo, Garrido, & Sánchez-Meca, 1997).

Attention deficit hyperactivity disorder

ADHD is characterized by reduced levels of concentration or attention, impulsivity, and overactivity or restlessness. There is no clear dividing line between extremes of normality and truly abnormal degrees of these behaviours.

Behavioural parenting approaches (i.e. approaches focused on modifying the child's behaviour) combined with advice to the child and teachers are effective for mild ADHD (Pfiffner, Yee Mikami, Huang-Pollock, Easterlin, Zalecki, & McBurnett, 2007). Where ADHD is more severe and impairing, a multimodal approach combining behavioural psychosocial interventions with children and parents, school consultation to help the child's teachers work with them effectively, and medication is effective (Jensen et al., 2007). Behaviour therapy alone is less effective than treatment with medicines known as psychostimulants (such as methylphenidate), which can help to bring hyperactive and aggressive behaviour under control. Behaviour therapy improves the ability to carry out instructions and complete tasks assigned and reduces disruptiveness, but this is unlikely to generalize beyond the classroom. In cases of impairing ADHD when medication cannot be monitored intensively, either a behavioural approach combining work with parents, child and school consultation, or standard medical care are effective.

It is unclear whether CBT is effective for ADHD, as the few available studies have reached different conclusions about this; it may be the behavioural component that is effective (Abikoff, 1991; Pliszka & AACAP Work Group on Quality Issues, 2007). More studies are needed in this area.

Social skills interventions that aim to foster cooperation and reciprocal exchange do not seem to improve peer relationships for children with ADHD, but, again, more studies are needed to confirm this (Cousins & Weiss, 1993).

We do not know whether systemic, psychodynamic or humanistic therapies are effective for ADHD, as this has not been systematically studied.

Tourette syndrome

Children and young people with Tourette syndrome experience repetitive and involuntary motor and vocal tics, such as blinking, shrugging or other more complex movements, or obscene language. The causes of these tics are not well understood.

Habit reversal (where the young person learns a response that is incompatible with the tic in order to stop themselves from performing it) seems to be an effective treatment for children and young people with Tourette syndrome and chronic motor tics (brief, uncontrollable, spasm-like movements) (Azrin & Peterson, 1990). There is no evidence for other behavioural treatments because this has not yet been the subject of significant research.

One study suggests that parent training may help to reduce disruptive behaviour in children with Tourette syndrome and ADHD, but further research is needed to confirm this (Scahill et al., 2006). Parent training appears ineffective in managing tics in children and young people with Tourette syndrome and chronic motor tics comorbid with ADHD.

Psychotic disorders

Schizophrenia	A long-term condition which may lead a person to believe that their false thought patterns are actually reality. Symptoms may include hallucinations, delusions and behavioural changes.
Bipolar disorder	This disorder is characterized by experience of extreme and long-lasting mood swings. Persons with the disorder have rotating periods of depression and mania, such that they can feel low and lethargic, but then euphoric and overactive.
Schizoaffective disorder	A mood disorder that combines bipolar disorder symptoms with psychotic symptoms. The disorder affects the mind such that patients may be confused as to reality and may experience hallucinations.

Findings from adult studies suggest that psychosocial treatment may be a promising line of approach to schizophrenia and bipolar disorder in children and young people, but too few studies have been done to enable any specific recommendations (Miklowitz, Biuckians, & Richards, 2006; Pavuluri, Graczyk, Henry, Carbray, Heidenreich, & Miklowitz, 2004). The only statement about psychosocial treatments for schizophrenia in children and young people that we can make with a degree of confidence is that cognitive remediation – a treatment which uses continuous behavioural exercises to boost memory power and attention – is ineffective (Pilling et al., 2002). There are a number of preliminary findings from single studies that require confirmation. It is possible that providing families with education about schizophrenia and working with them to reduce expressed emotion (criticism, hostility and emotional over-involvement) may reduce the need for later institutional care, although it is unlikely to influence relapse (Rund et al., 1994). An intervention described by the authors as 'supportive counselling' may be more acceptable, and therefore more effective, than CBT in reducing symptoms of schizophrenia in young people (Haddock, Lewis, Bentall, Dunn, Drake, & Tarrier, 2006). In this study both CBT and supportive counselling were carried out by the same five research therapists and the latter aimed to provide emotional support by developing a supportive relationship fostering rapport and unconditional regard for the client. Actively treating ongoing substance abuse and helping the young person to establish social networks may reduce the risk of disengagement with treatment.

It is possible that family interventions aimed at education, communication skills, stress reduction and problem-solving may reduce symptoms of bipolar disorder, but more research is needed to confirm this (Miklowitz et al., 2006).

There is no evidence of sufficiently high quality to allow us to make any statements about the effectiveness or otherwise of treatments for children and young people with schizoaffective disorder.

Pervasive developmental disorders

Pervasive developmental disorder (PDD)	The umbrella term used to denote disorders such as autism which involve delays in social skills such as communication and socialization.
Autism	A condition that affects how people perceive the social environment and interact with others. It is characterized by persistent problems in social communication and restrictive behaviours or interests.
Asperger's syndrome	Like autism, this is a condition that affects how people perceive the social environment and interact with others; however, it is not accompanied by learning difficulties and language skills may be higher.

Intensive behavioural treatment of young children with an autistic spectrum disorder (ASD) can improve their ability both to express themselves verbally and to listen to and understand others as well as their behaviour (Peters-Scheffer, Didden, Korzilius, & Sturmey, 2011). By this we mean that, with additional behavioural help, autistic children can be supported to convey their feelings with a greater degree of clarity, as well as participate with more confidence in peer exchanges. Our knowledge of how best to treat autism is, however, quite limited. Parent training may be helpful for children and young people with ASDs, but more research is needed (McConachie & Diggle, 2007). Similarly, one intervention, the Social Stories approach, which attempts to help the child to acquire social skills through the use of short, personalized stories to explain what happened or might happen in a particular situation, may be beneficial, but better designed studies are needed to confirm this (Karkhaneh, Clark, Ospina, Seida, Smith, & Hartling, 2010). Additionally, there is some evidence to suggest that CBT may be helpful for comorbid anxiety in children and young people with ASDs; however, more research is required (Chalfant, Rapee, & Carroll, 2007). There are no high-quality studies of sibling training, social skills training, video self-modelling, music therapy, self-management training, sensory integration therapy, or massage therapy for children and young people with ASDs. It is unclear whether educational interventions or courses teaching theory of mind are beneficial for children and young people with ASDs, as the available studies reach different conclusions about this and it is uncertain whether the benefits are lasting (Fisher & Happé, 2005; Ozonoff & Miller, 1995).

Social skills and problem-solving skills training, the Social Stories approach and CBT may be helpful for children with Asperger's syndrome, but more studies are needed (Sofronoff, Leslie, & Brown, 2004; Solomon, Goodlin-Jones, & Anders, 2004). CBT seems to be helpful for children with Asperger's and comorbid anxiety (Sofronoff, Attwood, & Hinton, 2005).

Self-injurious behaviour

Self-injurious behaviour (SIB) is increasingly common in young people. It is frequently associated with other difficulties, and many young people affected by it have a poor prognosis.

Brief hospital treatment seems to be helpful for young people with highly risky SIB (Hintikka, Marttunen, Pelkonen, Laukkanen, Viinamäki, & Lehtonen, 2006; Katz, Cox, Gunasekara, & Miller, 2004). No studies have directly compared inpatient treatment and home-based treatment of SIB, so we do not know which approach is more effective. It is possible that brief hospital admission may make it easier for the young person to attend outpatient treatment once they have been discharged.

It seems likely that engaging the young person effectively is necessary for treatment to succeed, although there is very little evidence directly linking effective engagement with better outcomes. Various approaches to help young people engage with treatment for SIB have been tested with some success, including negotiating treatment agreements, telephone follow-up after SIB, 'green cards' that act as passes to make it easier for the young person to be admitted to hospital if needed, and manualized 'therapeutic assessment' (Cotgrove, Zirinsky, Black, & Weston, 1995; Donaldson, Spirito, Arrigan, & Aspel, 1997). There is some evidence to suggest that manualized psychological treatments result in greater engagement and retention in treatment than TAU, but these results should be treated with caution, as there are numerous ways in which such results could be biased in favour of manualized treatments.

A few studies have looked at the effect of intensive treatment packages such as MST (home-based) and DBT (which can be delivered in various settings) on SIB (Huey et al., 2004; Rathus & Miller, 2002). MST (which involves a high proportion of family therapy) and ABFT have shown promise, but more research is needed (Diamond et al., 2010).

MST also involves intervening within the young person's wider social system. Although intuitively it may make sense that a cross-cutting intervention would be effective for tackling SIB, results for both MST and DBT have been mixed. Another systemic approach influenced by MST, the Youth-Nominated Support Team for Suicidal Adolescents (YST-1), was found to be no more effective than TAU (King, Kramer, Preuss, Kerr, Weisse, & Venkataraman, 2006).

Box 5.7   Dialectical behaviour therapy (DBT)

Dialectical behaviour therapy is based on CBT but also draws on Eastern philosophy and meditation practices and selected elements of other approaches, such as psychodynamic psychotherapy, client-centred counselling and gestalt. It encourages individuals to accept themselves as they are in the present and targets maladaptive behaviours by teaching skills of emotional regulation, core mindfulness, interpersonal effectiveness and distress tolerance.

There is hardly any research on whether or not individual CBT approaches to SIB are helpful, although problem-solving approaches have been highlighted as deserving further study. Group-based CBT and cognitive behavioural family therapy for SIB are no more effective than TAU, and group-based CBT is more expensive.

Mentalization-based treatment (a psychodynamic approach which involves individual and family treatment focused on the participants' capacity to understand their own and others' behaviour in order to reduce impulsive behaviour and help them to manage their feelings) may be an effective intervention for SIB in young people, especially where there is judged to be a risk of progression to borderline personality disorder. Given encouraging results from one trial by the programme developers, further research is warranted (Bleiberg, Roussow, & Fonagy, 2012).

Eating disorders

Anorexia	This is a mental health disorder where weight and shape concerns are driven by negative thoughts and feelings about the self. Characterized by severe weight loss, restrictive eating and compensatory behaviours, i.e. excessive exercise and/or self-induced vomiting.
Bulimia	Like anorexia nervosa, bulimia nervosa is characterized by restrictive eating and compensatory behaviours, i.e. excessive exercise and/or self-induced vomiting, however it differs in that people with bulimia typically maintain weight within the normal range due to recurrent cycles of binge eating and purging.

Anorexia

In situations where the young person is at serious physical risk, inpatient treatment is necessary. Although clinicians agree that specialist inpatient units are needed to treat anorexia, we do not know for sure what setting is best, as very few studies have looked at this. There is no clear evidence either for or against such specialist units (Gowers et al., 2010). Manualized family therapy is an effective treatment for anorexia (Lock, 2015). Even where there are high levels of family conflict, family therapy is still effective if the adolescent is seen separately from the parents (Lock & Gowers, 2005).

It is unclear whether or not manualized CBT is a helpful treatment for anorexia. Some studies have shown that family therapy achieves better results, but one study has found that CBT reduced the need for hospitalization compared to TAU (Gowers et al., 2010).

Bulimia

Manualized family therapy seems to be an effective treatment for young people with bulimia, and manualized individual CBT may also be effective (Le Grange, Lock, Agras, Bryson, & Jo, 2015). It is unclear whether family therapy or individual CBT produces better results with bulimic adolescents. One study found that in the short-term the individual approach was better, but by 12-month follow-up both treatments were equally effective (Schmidt et al., 2007).

Substance use disorders

The many forms of substance abuse, the difficulty of reaching or even identifying many young substance users, and the lack of trials with no-treatment control groups limit the generalizability of the conclusions we can draw from the available research. Given that many substance use disorders (SUDs) resolve spontaneously with age, the lack of such trials means we cannot say for sure that treatment is preferable to no treatment.

It is unclear whether specialist SUD services based in low-stigma settings or with outreach capacity produce better results than treatment integrated into generic child and adolescent mental health services (CAMHS), as this has not been studied systematically. Likewise, we do not know whether it is better to treat young people in outpatient or inpatient settings, as the available studies are of poor quality and reach different conclusions. Although we know that inpatients need active, ongoing follow-up post-discharge, we do not have enough evidence to know which of the available specific community outreach programmes are most effective.

Lower level substance abuse disorders

Brief CBT and motivational approaches, which support individuals to move beyond negative impulses for substance use by challenging harmful thought cycles, can prevent young people moving from low-level to serious use. In fact, when combined these two approaches tend to be more effective (Dennis et al., 2004). CBT often takes place in group settings, but we do not know how helpful the group setting might be; the number of studies is small and, while most suggest groups are effective, sometimes the results have been contradictory. There have been concerns that being in a group setting may make matters worse because the young people could have a negative influence on one another; however, there is no strong evidence to support these claims, as long as appropriate boundaries are maintained (Burleson, Kaminer, & Dennis, 2006).

Family/systemic therapy is a helpful treatment for lower level drug misuse; this approach can also be successful in combination with the use of CBT or motivational treatments (Austin, Macgowan, & Wagner, 2005; Latimer, Winters, D'Zurilla, & Nichols, 2003). Family/systems approaches can also help the young person to continue with their treatment and address other behavioural problems that often go hand-in-hand with SUD.

Although there is a well-established evidence base for 12-step programmes for treating adult addiction (i.e. Alcoholics Anonymous), we do not know whether or not an adapted version of this model for young people is effective, as there have been only a few studies with equivocal results (Kelly, Myers, & Brown, 2000).

Serious substance abuse disorders

Sadly, although our knowledge of effective interventions for SUDs continues to expand, we still do not know how best to identify and treat young people who are likely to have the worst outcomes; here, as across many other disorder domains, more research is needed.

A number of intensive programmes of treatment are available for SUDs that are particularly high risk, entrenched, or complex. These include MST, MDFT and the Adolescent Community Reinforcement Approach (A-CRA), a form of contingency management treatment which reinforces changes in behaviour with the aid of small prizes or tokens (Austin et al., 2005; Curtis, Ronan, & Borduin, 2004; Dennis et al., 2004). There are also briefer programmes that combine the use of CBT, motivational enhancement therapy and family therapy. All these treatment programmes may be effective in a meaningful number of cases, but more rigorous research is needed. In addition, we do not know whether any one particular programme is more effective than another, as the available studies have been conducted with very different groups and in very different settings.

Maltreatment

In this section we discuss treatments for the harmful effects of childhood maltreatment. The impact of maltreatment is wide-ranging, may be evident immediately or arise later, and the effects often endure into adulthood.

Physical and emotional abuse and neglect

Physical and emotional abuse and neglect can result in various kinds of emotional and behavioural difficulties. Among younger children, we have some evidence that group work focusing on developing cooperative and imaginative play can help with social and behavioural difficulties (Udwin, 1983). Violent delinquency in maltreated young people has been successfully reduced by a school-based violence prevention programme (Crooks, Scott, Wolfe, Chiodo, & Killip, 2007). CBT may be helpful for aggressive young people who have been physically abused (LeSure-Lester, 2002).

Exposure to interpersonal violence

Exposure to violence between parents or carers can result in PTSD, for which TF-CBT can be effective (Cohen, Mannarino, & Iyengar, 2011). PTSD in young children resulting from exposure to violence between parents and carers may be helped by child–parent psychotherapy. This is a specialist form of therapy which aims to foster a secure bond between parent and child following child trauma-exposure. One study found that providing mothers who had experienced intimate partner violence (IPV) with a safety plan and information about services available to them reduced the internalizing and externalizing behaviours of children exposed to the IPV (McFarlane, Groff, O'Brien, & Watson, 2005). Further work is needed to confirm these findings. Internalizing behaviours and harmful attitudes to violence can be improved by age-appropriate group work with children in a community setting to address their knowledge, attitudes and beliefs about family violence, their emotional adjustment and social behaviour, and externalizing behaviours are improved if this is supplemented by a parenting group (Graham-Bermann, Lynch, Banyard, DeVoe, & Halabu, 2007).

Sexual abuse

The effectiveness of treatments for children who have suffered sexual abuse has been quite widely investigated, and several meta-analyses of the available studies have found large to moderate **effect sizes**, which tend to be smaller in controlled studies. There is specific support from meta-analyses for psychotherapy (defined very broadly as any intervention designed to alleviate psychological distress, reduce maladaptive behaviour, or enhance adaptive behaviour through counselling, structured or unstructured interaction, a training programme or a predetermined treatment plan) (Harvey & Taylor, 2010), group treatment (Reeker, Ensing, & Elliott, 1997) and CBT combined with supportive, psychodynamic, or play therapy (Harvey & Taylor, 2010; Hetzel-Riggin, Brausch, & Montgomery, 2007; Sánchez-Meca, Rosa-Alcázar, & López-Soler, 2011). Play therapy, which enables children to process particular difficult events or emotions, does not seem to be effective when used on its own. In the case of the meta-analysis looking at psychotherapy, overall outcome and symptoms of PTSD were found to improve the most: moderate improvements were found for internalizing and externalizing symptoms, self-esteem and sexualized behaviour; and there were small to moderate improvements in coping and social skills. One meta-analysis, which looked at a range of treatments, found that longer treatments and more sessions produced larger effects, and older girls who had experienced sexual abuse within the family benefited more (Sánchez-Meca et al., 2011). In the case of group treatment, treatments that focused on the child only (compared to the child and their non-abusing parent) and those that lasted longer were both associated with larger effect sizes (Trask, Walsh, & Dilillo, 2011). Group treatment effects rose with age and were larger for the two studies that had a majority of boy participants (Trask et al., 2011).

CBT for the emotional and behavioural difficulties of sexually abused children – and specifically for anxiety – may be effective, although the available studies are not all of high quality (Macdonald et al., 2012). Group CBT with parallel parent work for sexual behaviour problems has a lasting effect (maintained at 10-year follow-up). TF-CBT including the mother and child may be effective for PTSD in sexually abused children (Cohen, Mannarino, & Knudsen, 2005). It is unclear whether or not CBT for depression in sexually abused children is helpful, as studies have reached different conclusions about this and a review found only a small effect size (Macdonald, Higgins, & Ramchandani, 2006).

It is possible that individual psychodynamic psychotherapy for sexually abused girls may help to relieve symptoms of depression, anxiety and PTSD (Trowell et al., 2002). More research is needed to confirm these suggestions.

Interventions for children with particular disorders following maltreatment

Group or individual CBT may be helpful for PTSD in maltreated children. EMDR therapy, an integrative psychotherapy designed specifically for trauma victims, and the anxiety medication propranolol may also be helpful (Ahmad, Larsson, & Sundelin-Wahlsten, 2007; Wethington et al., 2008). EMDR requires the patient to evoke an image of an event causing him or her anxiety, while tracking the therapist's finger as it is moved rapidly and rhythmically from side to side; at the same time, they generate cognitive coping statements. More research is needed to confirm these suggestions.

Interventions including parents to reduce the likelihood or recurrence of child maltreatment and improve the child's functioning

Parents whose children have been abused are difficult to engage and often drop out of treatment. PCIT, which draws on both attachment and social learning theory to foster supportive filial relations, can reduce parental maltreating behaviour and, to a limited extent, some of the child's difficulties. In preschool-age children, an attachment-based intervention which aims to demonstrate how the mother's personal history can affect her present-day relationship with her child, known as preschooler–parent psychotherapy, can help children who have developed harmfully negative ways of thinking about themselves and parent–child interactions (Toth, Maughan, Manly, Spagnola, & Cicchetti, 2002). Another very similar form of attachment-based psychotherapy – infant–parent psychotherapy – can increase rates of secure attachment among young children who have been maltreated (Cicchetti, Rogosch, & Toth, 2006). By this we mean that the process of therapy has enabled children who have previously been abused, and who are consequently very suspicious and afraid of adults, to successfully develop trusting and caring relationships with their primary caregivers. Overall, there is evidence in the form of several studies to support attachment-based interventions for maltreated young children and their carers, not only to increase attachment security, but also to reduce disorganized attachment, which is characterized by unpredictable behaviour, chronic mistrust of adults, lower levels of social competence and externalizing problems (Bernard, Dozier, Bick, Lewis-Morrarty, Lindhiem, & Carlson, 2012; Cicchetti et al., 2006; Moss, Dubois-Comtois, Cyr, Tarabulsy, St-Laurent, & Bernier, 2011).

MST can be effective in reducing parental maltreatment and improving the maltreated child's functioning (Swenson, Schaeffer, Henggeler, Faldowski, & Mayhew, 2010). Parent training and CBT are effective in reducing excessively harsh and abusive parenting. A psychoeducational parenting intervention addressing parenting skills, the mother's self-care and the fostering of adaptive competencies in the child may help to decrease young maltreated children's disorganized attachments (Cicchetti et al., 2006).

When it comes to interventions designed to reduce the likelihood of having to remove children from the family into foster care, treatments within family preservation programmes are unlikely to have any benefits (Dagenais, Begin, Bouchard, & Fortin, 2004; Littell & Schuerman, 1995). These preservation programmes are short-term, family-focused services for families in crisis, which aim to ensure that children can safely remain within their homes provided the parents receive additional assistance. Home visitation programmes also aim to ensure that the child does not have to be taken into an alternative care setting; however the evidence for their efficacy is rather mixed, with available studies reaching different conclusions (Macmillan, Wathen, Barlow, Fergusson, Levanthal, & Taussig, 2009).

When children are placed in foster care, it is imperative that they are not returned to their original family setting until their wellbeing and safety can be guaranteed. An intervention for maltreated children placed in foster care that involved assessment of parents and the parent–child interaction, and intensive work on these factors, succeeded in identifying parents who could not resume care of their children and reducing maltreatment of the children who returned to or remained with their parents, but was associated with longer stays in foster care (Zeanah et al., 2001). More research is needed to confirm the effectiveness of this approach.

Similarly, an intensive family reunification programme which emphasizes the necessity of support for family functioning, parenting and risk factors, may lead to a greater rate of rehabilitating children in foster care back to the home (Fraser, Walton, Lewis, Pecora, & Walton, 1996).

Change of caregiver as an intervention

Regular foster care does not reduce subsequent difficulties in fostered children compared to similar maltreated children who remain in the family home. Because children who are fostered are often very troubled, and it is not possible to randomly allocate them to foster care for research purposes, it is hard to measure how successful foster care can be, and we do not know whether regular foster care is better than leaving maltreated children at home, as the available studies have reached different conclusions. When children who remain in alternative care are compared with those who returned home, one study found that returning home was associated with poorer outcomes in terms of internalizing and externalizing behaviours, social adaptation, self-harm and educational progress (Taussig, Clyman, & Landsverk, 2001).

An attachment-based intervention, Attachment and Biobehavioral Catch-up, used with foster parents of very young children lowered the levels of the hormone cortisol in children's saliva (an indicator of stress) and reduced their behavioural problems (Bernard et al., 2012). The success of this intervention is likely to be down to its comprehensive design which, through weekly sessions, equipped carers with the skill-set to recognize child distress, nurture children's emotional expression and respond with warmth and affection irrespective of the child's behavioural problems.

For those in middle childhood in foster care, there is evidence that MTFC for the foster parents increases rates of successful placements (i.e. placements that do not break down), improves foster parents' ability to encourage and support the child's good behaviour, and reduces the child's behaviour problems. Two studies of MTFC have suggested that it may increase secure attachment and increase the rate of subsequent permanency of placement among preschool-age children, but more research is needed to confirm this (Fisher & Kim, 2007; Fisher, Burraston, & Pears, 2005).

The limits of our knowledge about what works for whom

As this review has shown, our knowledge about what works for whom is subject to some important limitations.

We know very little about appropriate treatment for a number of common conditions.

Box 5.8   Randomized controlled trials (RCTs) and their limitations

The great benefit of a RCT is that it enables the researcher or clinician to be more confident that the treatment was responsible for the outcomes observed, since, in principle, randomization ensures the even distribution of other factors that might affect the outcomes. While RCTs have often been thought of as the gold standard for a clinical trial, some caveats need to be kept in mind. A trial shows what can be achieved with a particular treatment under somewhat artificial conditions. The quality of the care available in the community may be different. People with multiple diagnoses are often excluded from trials and yet comorbidity is very common. Similarly, the common exclusion of those who cannot speak English means that the samples are often not representative of the communities they come from. By and large, RCTs are not designed to detect harmful effects of treatment. The results of RCTs are applied to less homogeneous populations with comorbidities, who are usually treated over longer periods of time, in clinical situations that at best vaguely resemble the cutting-edge clinical settings in which they were tested. Recognition of this issue has led reviewers to distinguish efficacy from effectiveness studies, with the second category more directly concerned with outcomes in a 'real world' practice setting (Seligman, 1996).

Indicators of a high-quality randomized controlled trial include:

- The study asks a clearly defined research question focused on the problem being studied.
- Randomization has been done in a way that ensures even distribution of known and unknown factors that might influence outcomes (**confounding variables**) and creates a control group that is as similar as possible to the treatment group. In smaller studies, special techniques such as **block randomization** and **stratification** may be needed to ensure that the size and characteristics of the groups are balanced.
- The researchers use **allocation concealment** techniques (such as use of a central telephone randomization service) to ensure that they do not know in advance who will be assigned to which group.
- Those responsible for collecting and analysing the data do not know who is in which group (this is known as '**blinding**').
- After randomization, it is usually the case that some people drop out of the study. Studies that analyse data from both treatment completers and study drop outs are regarded as of higher quality than studies that only consider treatment completers. This is known as **intention to treat analysis**.
- The sample size of the study is large enough to allow the study to detect a difference between the groups, if such a difference exists. This is referred to as the study's statistical power, as determined by its **power calculation**. If the study is not large enough, it is said to be underpowered and in this situation a finding of no difference may not be valid. Better quality studies will include discussion of the study's statistical power.

For a more detailed discussion, see (Akobeng, 2005).

More research is needed on subgroups of children and young people that are known to respond poorly to treatment. Even the most effective treatments are not effective for everyone who receives them. There is a need to investigate whether or not better results can be achieved with alternative methods.

Not all psychological treatments have been evaluated equally well. Systemic and psychodynamic psychotherapies are both widely provided in clinics, often when other, more evidence-based treatments have failed. Humanistic therapies and counselling are also very frequently offered. Research is urgently needed on whether some children in some situations might derive specific benefits from these approaches and what the effective elements are. It would be helpful to investigate whether components of these treatments could become part of an EBP protocol that clinicians could use in relation to particular clinical challenges. For example, managing ruptures in the treatment alliance (Safran, Muran, & Eubanks-Carter, 2011) could be helpful across a range of modalities.

Limitations of the available evidence

A number of limitations of the evidence base need to be taken into account. Too many 'evidence-based' interventions are backed up by just one or two studies. Studies conducted by researchers not involved in the development of the treatment which aim to replicate the results of the original studies are needed. To take a finding as 'fact' it must be supported by multiple independent studies, also known as 'replication studies'. Furthermore, the registration of all RCTs with the ISRCTN registry, the primary clinical trial registry recognized by WHO and the International Committee of Medical Journal Editors (ICMJE), and the publication of data from those trials, whether the outcomes are positive or negative, are essential if we are to interpret the evidence correctly.

Most published studies focus on symptoms and diagnoses as primary outcomes. However, to be truly effective, a treatment also needs to impact on other important areas, such as relationships with peers, family relationships, academic functioning and service utilization. When the focus is on diagnosis and/or symptoms, findings are inconsistent: some studies report complete remission of symptoms while others describe varying levels of reduction. Given the heterogeneity of many disorders and the clinical importance of sub-threshold cases, it is unwise to evaluate outcomes solely in terms of whether clients continue to meet criteria for a particular diagnosis.

Despite some improvements, too many reported studies still have significant methodological flaws. Sample sizes are often so small that studies are underpowered to find meaningful results. The bias towards publishing positive results from studies with small sample sizes leads to frequent failures of replication. Sample ages can also be a problem, with very wide age ranges reported in a sample and/or widely differing age of onset or time since onset of diagnosis within the sample. In depression research, large differences in outcome between clinically referred depressed young people and those recruited through advertisements have been reported, which are not attributable to greater severity. This indicates that even if an intervention is found to be effective in a study using a community population sample, this may not be the case for clinical patients. We must be cautious about extrapolating findings – especially, given that too many study samples still comprise non-distressed/non-referred participants.

Often studies have either no follow-up period or only a very brief one; as such we know very little about how long treatment should be continued once it has been shown to be effective. The value of intensive or extended psychological treatments and booster sessions has not been systematically evaluated in many contexts.

While it is now generally accepted that adverse effects of medication must be monitored and reported, this is rarely the case with psychological treatments, in which adverse events are almost universally assumed to be part of the presenting problem and associated difficult relationships and interactions. If psychological treatments can be beneficial, we can assume that they may also have the power to cause harm. Adverse outcome data have not been consistently collected or reported. For example, in studies of treatments for depression, it cannot be taken for granted that self-harm is a feature of the diagnosis rather than an adverse effect of treatment.

CBT has often been compared with therapies which, according to the criteria of Wampold (1997), are non bona fide (bona fide therapies are those with adequate therapist training, individualized treatment based on face-to-face meetings with the client, and inclusion of psychologically valid components). A meta-analysis by Spielmans, Pasek, & McFall (2007) attempted to identify the active ingredients in CBT for anxious and depressed children. The meta-analysis aggregated the results of studies in which CBT treatments were compared with other therapies. CBT was found to be significantly more effective than non bona fide treatments, but there was no evidence from direct comparisons to suggest that CBT was more efficacious than other bona fide treatments. There was only one comparison between CBT and a bona fide non-CBT treatment, which found that the two interventions were equally effective.

We often do not know how treatments that appear to be effective would compare with TAU in the real world when delivered by community clinicians to children with a variety of comorbid disorders. There are several reasons for this. Firstly, many well-designed trials compare new treatments with no-treatment control groups. Secondly, increasingly treatment trials have strict adherence guidelines to ensure we know exactly what has been delivered and evaluated, but this is not always easy to replicate in community settings. Manualized psychological treatments have become increasingly commercialized, which can mean that some evidence-based treatments are too expensive for services to adopt. Thirdly, while children with comorbid diagnoses are often excluded from treatment trials, comorbidity is the rule rather than the exception in community settings.

Box 5.9   How can we find out whether EBPs work in the real world?

To address our lack of knowledge about how apparently effective treatments compare with TAU in the real world, we need true **pragmatic trials** (i.e. taking place in usual clinical rather than specialized research settings) using quite simple protocols that are easy for practising clinicians to learn and deliver in community clinic settings. We also need to develop and evaluate effective methods to enable the delivery of effective treatments by community clinicians. Weisz, Doss and Hawley (2005) suggest that development of new interventions should take into account contextual variables such as characteristics of the practice setting. Under their deployment-focused model, development and evaluation of the intervention should take place in the context and with the clients who are representative of the intended application. EBPs should be part of an ongoing evolution of therapy, and routine practice settings should work with researchers to adapt interventions as appropriate to the context and evaluate these modifications (Garland, Plemmons, & Koontz, 2006).

We have seen that research has confirmed the effectiveness of a variety of multicomponent treatment packages for certain diagnoses. However, we do not know which elements of these packages are most helpful in particular clinical situations, and they are not usually compared against each other but instead tend to be compared to inactive conditions such as a wait-list control. We also do not know whether in some situations combinations of treatments may be more effective than individual treatments. In clinical practice, different treatments are more likely to be administered sequentially.

Box 5.10 A modular approach to psychological therapy

EBPs for depression, anxiety and conduct problems in young people produce mixed results in trials with the comorbid, complex cases seen in practice. In one study (Weisz et al., 2012) a multisite randomized effectiveness trial compared standard manualized treatment (one of three EBPs: CBT for depression, CBT for anxiety and behavioural parent training for conduct problems) with modular treatment allowing clinicians to use elements of the three separate treatment protocols more flexibly and with usual care. Eighty-four community clinicians were randomized to one of three conditions for the treatment of 174 clinically referred children aged 7–13. Outcomes were assessed using weekly youth and parent assessments. A standardized diagnostic assessment was also conducted before and after treatment. Modular treatment produced significantly steeper trajectories of improvement than usual care and standard treatment and youths receiving modular treatment also had significantly fewer diagnoses than youths receiving usual care after treatment. In contrast, outcomes of standard manualized treatment did not differ significantly from outcomes of usual care. The modular approach may be a promising way to build on the strengths of evidence-based treatments, improving their utility and effectiveness with referred youths in clinical practice settings.

Implications for clinical practice and research

We know that most conditions are under-recognized, that intervening earlier can reduce the risk of development of comorbid disorder, and that effective intervention can actually prevent subsequent episodes of disorder. Thus, there is an empirical case for early assessment and intervention services.

The available evidence on treatment for child mental health problems is based on standardized diagnostic criteria. Thus, it is important that treatment choice is informed by adequate diagnosis. However, given the high rates of comorbidity in child mental health disorders, clinicians will often need to decide which disorder(s) should be prioritized. A flexible approach is needed allowing for review, reassessment and further intervention as necessary. The resources of a multidisciplinary team are likely to be required to enable this to happen. In a school setting this may involve routine liaison between the school counsellor and Special Educational Needs Co-ordinator (SENCO), with additional input from external service support when required.

There is consistent evidence across disorders that benefits for the child are associated with the direct involvement of family and/or caregivers in assessment and appropriate therapeutic intervention. Children also benefit more when information is routinely sought from agencies such as schools and social services that are also involved with the child and family (Kazak et al., 2010). CAMHS should be designed to enable well-integrated multi-agency involvement, with good communication between the different agencies. Research is needed to determine the service context and the characteristics of individual therapists best placed to engage hard-to-reach families with multiple problems, particularly in families where there is or has been child maltreatment, substance misuse and/or conduct disorder.

We need to be mindful of the risk that the rise of certain well-publicized evidence-based interventions will stifle innovation. It is important that services are able to deliver EBPs, but such interventions will never work for everyone. We need to be able to develop alternative interventions alongside existing evidence-based approaches to mitigate the risk of complacency or offering interventions that are not as helpful to children and young people as they could be.

Conclusion

A great deal of work needs to be done to make psychological treatments genuinely accessible. The proportion of children and young people who need mental health interventions is increasing, while the availability of resources for interventions is not keeping pace and may even be on the decline (Kazdin & Blase, 2011). Current specialist CAMHS provide insufficient access for a large proportion of the children who need them. New sustainable models of delivery are needed.

A genuinely ecologically sound mental health service for children and young people will require the empowerment of communities, schools, peers and families, as well as the child, to deliver evidence-based services in healthcare delivery structures and other contexts that are safe, resilience-enhancing and readily accessible.

We need to stop pretending that psychotherapy is like a chemical carefully purified in the laboratory, distinct from the millions of other molecules which we come across in our day-to-day lives. Therapy is a social experience and as such is best integrated with all the other social experiences which help us navigate life's ups and downs: education, sport, peer relationships, music and theatre, to name but a few. Psychological therapy should be integrated with the rest of a child's life, not removed from it, if it is to generalize and to change behaviour and experience in all these contexts.

The next generation of therapies will be preventive and resilience-building; positive as opposed to symptom-focused. As the principles of psychological and brain development become clearer to science, the application of these principles to the encouragement of healthy development has the potential to reduce the prevalence of distress and increase the proportion of young people who go through life without a diagnosis of mental disorder.

Recommended reading

Fonagy, P., Cottrell, D., Phillips, J., Bevington, D., Glaser, D., & Allison, E. (2014). *What works for whom? A critical review of treatments for children and adolescents* (2nd ed.). New York: Guilford Press. This book provides a comprehensive review of the evidence base for both physical and psychological treatments for mental health disorders in children and young people.

Questions for reflection

- Did any of the findings presented in this review surprise you? Why?
- In which of the areas of uncertainty identified above do you feel it would be most important to conduct further research?
- In what ways could you use the findings presented here to inform your clinical practice?

References

Abikoff, H. (1991). Cognitive training in ADHD children: Less to it than meets the eye. *Journal of Learning Disabilities*, 24, 205–209.

Ahmad, A., Larsson, B., & Sundelin-Wahlsten, V. (2007). EMDR treatment for children with PTSD: Results of a randomized controlled trial. *Nordic Journal of Psychiatry*, 61, 349–354.

Ahrens, J., & Rexford, L. (2002). Cognitive processing therapy for incarcerated adolescents with PTSD. *Journal of Aggression, Maltreatment and Trauma*, 6, 201–216.

Akobeng, A. K. (2005). Understanding randomised controlled trials. *Archives of Disease in Childhood*, 90, 840–844.

American Psychiatric Association. (1994). *Diagnostic and statistical manual of mental disorders* (4th ed.). Washington, DC: American Psychiatric Association.

American Psychiatric Association. (2013). *Diagnostic and statistical manual of mental disorders* (5th ed.). Washington, DC: American Psychiatric Association.

Andrews, D. A., & Bonta, J. (2006). *The psychology of criminal conduct* (4th ed.). Newark, NJ: LexisNexis/Matthew Bender.

APA Presidential Task Force on Evidence-Based Practice. (2006). Evidence-based practice in psychology. *American Psychologist*, 61, 271–285.

Austin, A. M., Macgowan, M. J., & Wagner, E. F. (2005). Effective family-based interventions for adolescents with substance use problems: A systematic review. *Research on Social Work Practice*, 15, 67–83.

Azrin, N. H., & Peterson, A. L. (1990). Treatment of Tourette syndrome by habit reversal: A waiting list control group comparison. *Behavior Therapy*, 21, 305–318.

Bandoroff, S., & Scherer, D. G. (1994). Wilderness family therapy: An innovative treatment approach for problem youth. *Journal of Child and Family Studies*, 3, 175–191.

Barbe, R. P., Bridge, J. A., Birmaher, B., Kolko, D. J., & Brent, D. A. (2004). Lifetime history of sexual abuse, clinical presentation, and outcome in a clinical trial for adolescent depression. *Journal of Clinical Psychiatry*, 65, 77–83.

Barrington, J., Prior, M., Richardson, M., & Allen, K. (2005). Effectiveness of CBT versus standard treatment for childhood anxiety disorders in a community clinic setting. *Behaviour Change*, 22, 29–43.

Beardslee, W. R., Brent, D. A., Weersing, V. R., Clarke, G. N., Porta, G., Hollon, S. D., . . . Garber, J. (2013). Prevention of depression in at-risk adolescents: Longer-term effects. *JAMA Psychiatry*, 70, 1161–1170.

Beidel, D. C., Turner, S. M., Sallee, F. R., Ammerman, R. T., Crosby, L. A., & Pathak, S. (2007). SET-C versus fluoxetine in the treatment of childhood social phobia. *Journal of the American Academy of Child and Adolescent Psychiatry*, 46, 1622–1632.

Beidel, D. C., Turner, S. M., & Young, B. J. (2006). Social effectiveness therapy for children: Five years later. *Behavior Therapy*, 37, 416–425.

Bennett, D. S., & Gibbons, T. A. (2000). Efficacy of child cognitive-behavioral interventions for antisocial behavior: A meta-analysis. *Child & Family Behavior Therapy*, 22, 1–15.

Bernard, K., Dozier, M., Bick, J., Lewis-Morrarty, E., Lindhiem, O., & Carlson, E. (2012). Enhancing attachment organization among maltreated children: Results of a randomized clinical trial. *Child Development*, 83, 623–636.

Biegel, G. M., Brown, K. W., Shapiro, S. L., & Schubert, C. M. (2009). Mindfulness-based stress reduction for the treatment of adolescent psychiatric outpatients: A randomized clinical trial. *Journal of Consulting and Clinical Psychology*, 77, 855–866.

Biehal, N., Ellison, S., & Sinclair, I. (2011). Intensive fostering: An independent evaluation of MTFC in an English setting. *Children and Youth Services Review*, 33, 2043–2049.

Birmaher, B., Brent, D. A., Kolko, D., Baugher, M., Bridge, J., Holder, D., Iyengar. S., & Ulloa, R. E. (2000). Clinical outcome after short-term psychotherapy for adolescents with major depressive disorder. *Archives of General Psychiatry*, 57, 29–36.

Bleiberg, E., Roussow, T., & Fonagy, P. (2012). Adolescent breakdown and emerging borderline personality disorder. In A. W. Bateman & P. Fonagy (Eds.), *Handbook of mentalizing in mental health practice* (pp. 463–510). Arlington, VA: American Psychiatric Publishing.

Bolton, D., Williams, T., Perrin, S., Atkinson, L., Gallop, C., Waite, P., & Salkovskis, P. (2011). Randomized controlled trial of full and brief cognitive-behaviour therapy and wait-list for paediatric obsessive-compulsive disorder. *Journal of Child Psychology and Psychiatry*, 52, 1269–1278.

Brent, D. A., Holder, D., Kolko, D., Birmaher, B., Baugher, M., Roth, C., Iyengar, S., & Johnson, B. A. (1997). A clinical psychotherapy trial for adolescent depression comparing cognitive, family, and supportive therapy. *Archives of General Psychiatry*, 54, 877–885.

Burleson, J. A., Kaminer, Y., & Dennis, M. L. (2006). Absence of iatrogenic or contagion effects in adolescent group therapy: Findings from the Cannabis Youth Treatment (CYT) study. *American Journal on Addictions*, 15 (Suppl. 1), 4–15.

Cartwright-Hatton, S., Roberts, C., Chitsabesan, P., Fothergill, C., & Harrington, R. (2004). Systematic review of the efficacy of cognitive behaviour therapies for childhood and adolescent anxiety disorders. *British Journal of Clinical Psychology*, 43(Pt 4), 421–436.

Cary, C. E., & McMillen, J. C. (2012). The data behind the dissemination: A systematic review of trauma-focused cognitive behavioral therapy for use with children and youth. *Children and Youth Services Review*, 34, 748–757.

Chalfant, A. M., Rapee, R., & Carroll, L. (2007). Treating anxiety disorders in children with high functioning autism spectrum disorders: A controlled trial. *Journal of Autism and Developmental Disorders*, 37, 1842–1857.

Cicchetti, D., Rogosch, F. A., & Toth, S. L. (2006). Fostering secure attachment in infants in maltreating families through preventive interventions. *Development and Psychopathology*, 18, 623–649.

Clarke, G. N., Lewinsohn, P. M., & Hops, H. (1990). Leader's manual for adolescent groups. Adolescent Coping With Depression course. Retrieved from www.kpchr.org/research/public/common/getdocpublic.aspx?docid = 53468A11-CDDF-4E20-A98F-9EEA4DE94C39

Clarke, G. N., Rohde, P., Lewinsohn, P. M., Hops, H., & Seeley, J. R. (1999). Cognitive-behavioral treatment of adolescent depression: Efficacy of acute group treatment and booster sessions. *Journal of the American Academy of Child and Adolescent Psychiatry*, 38, 272–279.

Cobham, V. E., Dadds, M. R., & Spence, S. H. (1998). The role of parental anxiety in the treatment of childhood anxiety. *Journal of Consulting and Clinical Psychology*, 66, 893–905.

Cohen, J. A., Mannarino, A. P., & Iyengar, S. (2011). Community treatment of posttraumatic stress disorder for children exposed to intimate partner violence: A randomized controlled trial. *Archives of Pediatrics and Adolescent Medicine*, 165, 16–21.

Cohen, J. A., Mannarino, A. P., & Knudsen, K. (2005). Treating sexually abused children: 1 year follow-up of a randomized controlled trial. *Child Abuse & Neglect*, 29, 135–145.

Cotgrove, A. J., Zirinsky, L., Black, D., & Weston, D. (1995). Secondary prevention of attempted suicide in adolescence. *Journal of Adolescence*, 18, 569–577.

Cousins, L. S., & Weiss, G. (1993). Parent training and social skills training for children with attention-deficit hyperactivity disorder: How can they be combined for greater effectiveness? *Canadian Journal of Psychiatry*, 38, 449–457.

Cox, G. R., Callahan, P., Churchill, R., Hunot, V., Merry, S. N., Parker, A. G., & Hetrick, S. E. (2014). Psychological therapies versus antidepressant medication, alone and in combination for depression in children and adolescents. *Cochrane Database of Systematic Reviews*, 11, CD008324.

Crooks, C. V., Scott, K. L., Wolfe, D. A., Chiodo, D., & Killip, S. (2007). Understanding the link between childhood maltreatment and violent delinquency: What do schools have to add? *Child Maltreatment*, 12, 269–280.

Curtis, N. M., Ronan, K. R., & Borduin, C. M. (2004). Multisystemic treatment: A meta-analysis of outcome studies. *Journal of Family Psychology*, 18, 411–419.

Cuthbert, B. N., & Insel, T. R. (2013). Toward the future of psychiatric diagnosis: The seven pillars of RDoC. *BMC Medicine*, 11, 126.

Dagenais, C., Begin, J., Bouchard, C., & Fortin, D. (2004). Impact of intensive family support programs: A synthesis of evaluation studies. *Children and Youth Services Review*, 26, 249–263.

Daleiden, E. L., & Chorpita, B. F. (2005). From data to wisdom: Quality improvement strategies supporting large-scale implementation of evidence-based services. *Child and Adolescent Psychiatric Clinics of North America*, 14, 329–349.

De Cuyper, S., Timbremont, B., Braet, C., De Backer, V., & Wullaert, T. (2004). Treating depressive symptoms in schoolchildren: A pilot study. *European Child & Adolescent Psychiatry*, 13, 105–114.

Dennis, M., Godley, S. H., Diamond, G., Tims, F. M., Babor, T., Donaldson, J., Liddle, H., Titus, J. C., Kaminer, Y., Webb, C., Hamilton, N., & Funk, R. (2004). The Cannabis Youth Treatment (CYT) Study: Main findings from two randomized trials. *Journal of Substance Abuse Treatment*, 27, 197–213.

Diamond, G. S., Wintersteen, M. B., Brown, G. K., Diamond, G. M., Gallop, R., Shelef, K., & Levy, S. (2010). Attachment-based family therapy for adolescents with suicidal ideation: A randomized controlled trial. *Journal of the American Academy of Child and Adolescent Psychiatry*, 49, 122–131.

Dishion, T. J., & Andrews, D. W. (1995). Preventing escalation in problem behaviors with high-risk young adolescents: Immediate and 1-year outcomes. *Journal of Consulting and Clinical Psychology*, 63, 538–548.

Dishion, T. J., & Kavanagh, K. (2003). *Intervening in adolescent problem behavior: A family-centered approach*. New York: Guilford Press.

Donaldson, D., Spirito, A., Arrigan, M., & Aspel, J. W. (1997). Structured disposition planning for adolescent suicide attempters in a general hospital: Preliminary findings on short-term outcome. *Archives of Suicide Research*, 3, 271–82.

Drake, E. K., & Barnoski, R. (2006). *Recidivism findings for the Juvenile Rehabilitation Administration's dialectical behavior therapy program: Final report*. Olympia, WA: Washington State Institute for Public Policy.

Drugli, M. B., Larsson, B., Fossum, S., & Morch, W. T. (2010). Five- to six-year outcome and its prediction for children with ODD/CD treated with parent training. *Journal of Child Psychology and Psychiatry*, 51, 559–566.

Ertl, V., Pfeiffer, A., Schauer, E., Elbert, T., & Neuner, F. (2011). Community-implemented trauma therapy for former child soldiers in Northern Uganda: A randomized controlled trial. *Journal of the American Medical Association*, 306, 503–512.

Farrington, D. P., & Ttofi, M. M. (2009). Reducing school bullying: Evidence-based implications for policy. *Crime and Justice*, 38, 281–345.

Fernandez, M. A., & Eyberg, S. M. (2009). Predicting treatment and follow-up attrition in parent–child interaction therapy. *Journal of Abnormal Child Psychology*, 37, 431–441.

Field, A., & Cottrell, D. (2011). Eye movement desensitization and reprocessing as a therapeutic intervention for traumatized children and adolescents: A systematic review of the evidence for family therapists. *Journal of Family Therapy*, 33, 374–388.

Fisher, N., & Happé, F. (2005). A training study of theory of mind and executive function in children with autistic spectrum disorders. *Journal of Autism and Developmental Disorders*, 35, 757–771.

Fisher, P. A., & Kim, H. K. (2007). Intervention effects on foster preschoolers' attachment-related behaviors from a randomized trial. *Prevention Science*, 8, 161–170.

Fisher, P. A., Burraston, B., & Pears, K. (2005). The early intervention foster care program: Permanent placement outcomes from a randomized trial. *Child Maltreatment*, 10, 61–71.

Forgatch, M. S., & Ramsey, E. (1994). Boosting homework: A video tape link between families and schools. *School Psychology Review*, 23, 472–484.

Fraser, M. W., Walton, E., Lewis, R. E., Pecora, P. J., & Walton, W. K. (1996). An experiment in family reunification: Correlates of outcomes at one-year follow-up. *Children and Youth Services Review*, 18, 335–361.

Fristad, M. A., Verducci, J. S., Walters, K., & Young, M. E. (2009). Impact of multifamily psychoeducational psychotherapy in treating children aged 8 to 12 years with mood disorders. *Archives of General Psychiatry*, 66, 1013–1021.

Galla, B. M., Wood, J. J., Chiu, A. W., Langer, D. A., Jacobs, J., Ifekwunigwe, M., & Larkins, C. (2012). One year follow-up to modular cognitive behavioral therapy for the treatment of pediatric anxiety disorders in an elementary school setting. *Child Psychiatry and Human Development*, 43, 219–226.

Garcia, A. M., Sapyta, J. J., Moore, P. S., Freeman, J. B., Franklin, M. E., March, J. S., & Foa, E. B. (2010). Predictors and moderators of treatment outcome in the Pediatric Obsessive Compulsive Treatment Study (POTS I). *Journal of the American Academy of Child and Adolescent Psychiatry*, 49, 1024–1033.

Garland, A., Plemmons, D., & Koontz, L. (2006). Research-practice parternship in mental health: Lessons from participants. *Administration and Policy in Mental Health*, 33, 517–528.

Ghosh Ippen, C., Harris, W. W., Van Horn, P., & Lieberman, A. F. (2011). Traumatic and stressful events in early childhood: Can treatment help those at highest risk? *Child Abuse & Neglect*, 35, 504–513.

Goodyer, I. M., Dubicka, B., Wilkinson, P., Kelvin, R., Roberts, C., Byford, S., . . . Harrington, R. (2008). A randomised controlled trial of cognitive behaviour therapy in adolescents with major depression treated by selective serotonin reuptake inhibitors. The ADAPT trial. *Health Technology Assessment*, 12, iii–iv, ix–60.

Gowers, S. G., Clark, A. F., Roberts, C., Byford, S., Barrett, B., Griffiths, A., Edwards, V., Bryan, C., Smethurst, N., Rowlands, L., & Roots, P. (2010). A randomised controlled multicentre trial of treatments for adolescent anorexia nervosa including assessment of cost-effectiveness and patient acceptability: The TOuCAN trial. *Health Technology Assessment*, 14, 1–98.

Graham-Bermann, S. A., Lynch, S., Banyard, V., DeVoe, E. R., & Halabu, H. (2007). Community-based intervention for children exposed to intimate partner violence: An efficacy trial. *Journal of Consulting and Clinical Psychology*, 75, 199–209.

Gunlicks-Stoessel, M., Mufson, L., Jekal, A., & Turner, J. B. (2010). The impact of perceived interpersonal functioning on treatment for adolescent depression: IPT-A versus treatment as usual in school-based health clinics. *Journal of Consulting and Clinical Psychology*, 78, 260–267.

Haddock, G., Lewis, S., Bentall, R., Dunn, G., Drake, R., & Tarrier, N. (2006). Influence of age on outcome of psychological treatments in first-episode psychosis. *British Journal of Psychiatry*, 188, 250–254.

Harper, N. J., & Russell, K. C. (2008). Family involvement and outcome in adolescent wilderness treatment: A mixed-methods evaluation. *International Journal of Child and Family Welfare*, 11, 19–36.

Harvey, S. T., & Taylor, J. E. (2010). A meta-analysis of the effects of psychotherapy with sexually abused children and adolescents. *Clinical Psychology Review*, 30, 517–535.

Hetzel-Riggin, M. D., Brausch, A. M., & Montgomery, B. S. (2007). A meta-analytic investigation of therapy modality outcomes for sexually abused children and adolescents: An exploratory study. *Child Abuse & Neglect*, 31, 125–141.

Hintikka, U., Marttunen, M., Pelkonen, M., Laukkanen, E., Viinamäki, H., & Lehtonen, J. (2006). Improvement in cognitive and psychosocial functioning and self image among adolescent inpatient suicide attempters. *BMC Psychiatry*, 6, 58.

Huey, S. J., Henggeler, S. W., Rowland, M. D., Halliday-Boykins, C. A., Cunningham, P. B., Pickrel, S. G., & Edwards, J. (2004). Multisystemic therapy effects on attempted suicide by youths presenting psychiatric emergencies. *Journal of the American Academy of Child and Adolescent Psychiatry*, 43, 183–190.

Hutchings, J., Bywater, T., Williams, M. E., Whitaker, C., Lane, E., & Shakespeare, K. (2011). The extended school aged Incredible Years parent program. *Child and Adolescent Mental Health*, 16, 136–143.

In-Albon, T., & Schneider, S. (2007). Psychotherapy of childhood anxiety disorders: A meta-analysis. *Psychotherapy and Psychosomatics*, 76, 15–24.

Ishikawa, S. I., Okajima, I., Matsuoka, H., & Sakano, Y. (2007). Cognitive behavioural therapy for anxiety disorders in children and adolescents: A meta-analysis. *Child and Adolescent Mental Health*, 12, 164–172.

James, A., Soler, A., & Weatherall, R. (2005). Cognitive behavioural therapy for anxiety disorders in children and adolescents. *Cochrane Database of Systematic Reviews*, 4, CD004690.

Jensen, P. S., Arnold, L. E., Swanson, J. M., Vitiello, B., Abikoff, H. B., Greenhill, L. L., . . . Hur, K. (2007). 3-year follow-up of the NIMH MTA study. *Journal of the American Academy of Child and Adolescent Psychiatry*, 46, 989–1002.

Kahle, A. L., & Kelley, M. L. (1994). Children's homework problems: A comparison of goal setting and parent training. *Behaviour Therapy*, 25, 275–290.

Karkhaneh, M., Clark, B., Ospina, M. B., Seida, J. C., Smith, V., & Hartling, L. (2010). Social Stories to improve social skills in children with autism spectrum disorder: A systematic review. *Autism*, 14, 641–662.

Kataoka, S. H., Stein, B. D., Jaycox, L. H., Wong, M., Escudero, P., Tu, W., . . . Fink, A. (2003). A school-based mental health program for traumatized Latino immigrant children. *Journal of the American Academy of Child and Adolescent Psychiatry*, 42, 311–318.

Katz, L. Y., Cox, B. J., Gunasekara, S., & Miller, A. L. (2004). Feasibility of dialectical behavior therapy for suicidal adolescent inpatients. *Journal of the American Academy of Child and Adolescent Psychiatry*, 43, 276–282.

Kazak, A. E., Hoagwood, K., Weisz, J. R., Hood, K., Kratochwill, T. R., Vargas, L. A., & Banez, G. A. (2010). A meta-systems approach to evidence-based practice for children and adolescents. *American Psychologist*, 65, 85–97.

Kazdin, A. E. (1997). Parent management training: Evidence, outcomes, and issues. *Journal of the American Academy of Child and Adolescent Psychiatry*, 36, 1349–1356.

Kazdin, A. E. (2010). Problem-solving skills training and parent management training for oppositional defiant disorder and conduct disorder. In A. E. Kazdin & J. R. Weisz (Eds.), *Evidence-based psychotherapies for children and adolescents* (pp. 211–226). New York: Guilford Press.

Kazdin, A. E., & Blase, S. L. (2011). Rebooting psychotherapy research and practice to reduce the burden of mental illness. *Perspectives on Psychological Science*, 6, 21–37.

Kazdin, A. E., & Wassell, G. (2000). Predictors of barriers to treatment and therapeutic change in outpatient therapy for antisocial children and their families. *Mental Health Services Research*, 2, 27–40.

Kazdin, A. E., & Whitley, M. K. (2006). Comorbidity, case complexity, and effects of evidence-based treatment for children referred for disruptive behavior. *Journal of Consulting and Clinical Psychology*, 74, 455–467.

Kelly, J. F., Myers, M. G., & Brown, S. A. (2000). A multivariate process model of adolescent 12-step attendance and substance use outcome following inpatient treatment. *Psychology of Addictive Behaviors*, 14, 376–389.

Kendall, P. C. (1994). Treating anxiety disorders in children: Results of a randomized clinical trial. *Journal of Consulting and Clinical Psychology*, 62, 100–110.

Kendall, P. C., Hudson, J. L., Gosch, E., Flannery-Schroeder, E., & Suveg, C. (2008). Cognitive-behavioral therapy for anxiety disordered youth: A randomized clinical trial evaluating child and family modalities. *Journal of Consulting and Clinical Psychology*, 76, 282–297.

Kendall, P. C., Safford, S., Flannery-Schroeder, E., & Webb, A. (2004). Child anxiety treatment: Outcomes in adolescence and impact on substance use and depression at 7.4-year follow-up. *Journal of Consulting and Clinical Psychology*, 72, 276–287.

King, C. A., Kramer, A., Preuss, L., Kerr, D. C. R., Weisse, L., & Venkataraman, S. (2006). Youth-Nominated Support Team for Suicidal Adolescents (Version 1): A randomized controlled trial. *Journal of Consulting and Clinical Psychology*, 74, 199–206.

Kroll, L., Harrington, R., Jayson, D., Fraser, J., & Gowers, S. (1996). Pilot study of continuation cognitive-behavioral therapy for major depression in adolescent psychiatric patients. *Journal of the American Academy of Child and Adolescent Psychiatry*, 35, 1156–1161.

Landenberger, N. A., & Lipsey, M. W. (2005). The positive effects of cognitive-behavioral programs for offenders: A meta-analysis of factors associated with effective treatment. *Journal of Experimental Criminology*, 1, 451–476.

Last, C. G., Hansen, C., & Franco, N. (1998). Cognitive-behavioral treatment of school phobia. *Journal of the American Academy of Child and Adolescent Psychiatry*, 37, 404–411.

Latimer, W. W., Winters, K. C., D'Zurilla, T., & Nichols, M. (2003). Integrated family and cognitive-behavioral therapy for adolescent substance abusers: A stage I efficacy study. *Drug and Alcohol Dependence*, 71, 303–317.

Lau, W. Y., Chan, C. K., Li, J. C., & Au, T. K. (2010). Effectiveness of group cognitive-behavioral treatment for childhood anxiety in community clinics. *Behaviour Research and Therapy*, 48, 1067–1077.

Le Grange, D., Lock, J., Agras, W. S., Bryson, S. W., & Jo, B. (2015). Randomized clinical trial of family-based treatment and cognitive-behavioral therapy for adolescent bulimia nervosa. *Journal of the American Academy of Child and Adolescent Psychiatry*, 54, 886–894 e2.

Lenze, S. N., Pautsch, J., & Luby, J. (2011). Parent–child interaction therapy emotion development: A novel treatment for depression in preschool children. *Depression and Anxiety*, 28, 153–159.

LeSure-Lester, G. E. (2002). An application of cognitive-behavior principles in the reduction of aggression among abused African American adolescents. *Journal of Interpersonal Violence*, 17, 394–402.

Lewin, A. B., Storch, E. A., Geffken, G. R., Goodman, W. K., & Murphy, T. K. (2006). A neuropsychiatric review of pediatric obsessive-compulsive disorder: Etiology and efficacious treatments. *Neuropsychiatric Disease and Treatment*, 2, 21–31.

Liber, J. M., Van Widenfelt, B. M., Utens, E. M., Ferdinand, R. F., Van der Leeden, A. J., Van Gastel, W., & Treffers, P. D. (2008). No differences between group versus individual treatment of childhood anxiety disorders in a randomised clinical trial. *Journal of Child Psychology and Psychiatry*, 49, 886–893.

Liddle, H. A., Dakof, G. A., Henderson, C., & Rowe, C. (2011). Implementation outcomes of multidimensional family therapy-detention to community: A reintegration program for drug-using juvenile detainees. *International Journal of Offender Therapy and Comparative Criminology*, 55, 587–604.

Liddle, H. A., Dakof, G. A., Turner, R. M., Henderson, C. E., & Greenbaum, P. E. (2008). Treating adolescent drug abuse: A randomized trial comparing multidimensional family therapy and cognitive behavior therapy. *Addiction*, 103, 1660–1670.

Lieberman, A. F., Van Horn, P., & Ghosh Ippen, C. (2005). Toward evidence-based treatment: Child–parent psychotherapy with preschoolers exposed to marital violence. *Journal of the American Academy of Child and Adolescent Psychiatry*, 44, 1241–1248.

Lipsey, M. W. (2009). The primary factors that characterize effective interventions with juvenile offenders: A meta-analytic overview. *Victims & Offenders*, 4, 124–147.

Lipsey, M. W., Landenberger, N. A., & Wilson, S. J. (2007). Effects of cognitive-behavioral programs for criminal offenders. *Campbell Systematic Reviews 2007*, 6.

Littell, J. H., & Schuerman, J. R. (1995). *A synthesis of research on family preservation and family reunification programs*. Rockville, MD: Westat.

Lochman, J. E., & Wells, K.C. (2003). Effectiveness study of Coping Power and classroom intervention with aggressive children: Outcomes at one year follow-up. *Behavior Therapy*, 34, 493–515.

Lochman, J. E., & Wells, K. C. (2004). The Coping Power program for preadolescent aggressive boys and their parents: Outcome effects at the 1-year follow-up. *Journal of Consulting and Clinical Psychology, 72,* 571–578.

Lochman, J. E., Boxmeyer, C., Powell, N. P., Barry, T. D., & Pardini, D. A. (2010). Anger control training in aggressive youths. In A. E. Kazdin & J. R. Weisz (Eds.), *Evidence-based psychotherapies for children and adolescents* (pp. 227–242). New York: Guilford Press.

Lochman, J. E., Wells, K., & Lenhart, L. (2008). *Coping Power: Child group facilitator's guide.* New York: Oxford University Press

Lock, J. (2015). An update on evidence-based psychosocial treatments for eating disorders in children and adolescents. *Journal of Clinical Child & Adolescent Psychology, 44*(5), 707–21.

Lock, J., & Gowers, S. (2005). Effective interventions for adolescents with anorexia nervosa. *Journal of Mental Health, 14,* 599–610.

Lundahl, B., Risser, H. J., & Lovejoy, M. C. (2006). A meta-analysis of parent training: Moderators and follow-up effects. *Clinical Psychology Review, 26,* 86–104.

Lusk, P., & Melnyk, B. M. (2011). COPE for the treatment of depressed adolescents: Lessons learned from implementing an evidence-based practice change. *Journal of the American Psychiatric Nurses Association, 17,* 297–309.

Macdonald, G. M., Higgins, J. P., & Ramchandani, P. (2006). Cognitive-behavioural interventions for children who have been sexually abused. *Cochrane Database of Systematic Reviews,* 4, CD001930.

Macdonald, G., Higgins, J. P., Ramchandani, P., Valentine, J. C., Bronger, L. P., Klein, P., . . . Taylor, M. (2012). Cognitive-behavioural interventions for children who have been sexually abused. *Cochrane Database of Systematic Reviews,* 5, CD001930.

Macmillan, H. L., Wathen, C. N., Barlow, J., Fergusson, D. M., Leventhal, J. M., & Taussig, H. N. (2009). Interventions to prevent child maltreatment and associated impairment. *Lancet, 373,* 250–266.

Manassis, K., Mendlowitz, S. L., Scapillato, D., Avery, D., Fiksenbaum, L., Freire, M., . . . Owens, M. (2002). Group and individual cognitive-behavioral therapy for childhood anxiety disorders: *Journal of the American Academy of Child and Adolescent Psychiatry, 41,* 1423–1430.

McCart, M. R., Priester, P. E., Davies, W. H., & Azen, R. (2006). Differential effectiveness of behavioral parent-training and cognitive-behavioral therapy for antisocial youth: A meta-analysis. *Journal of Abnormal Child Psychology, 34,* 527–543.

McConachie, H., & Diggle, T. (2007). Parent implemented early intervention for young children with autism spectrum disorder: A systematic review. *Journal of Evaluation in Clinical Practice, 13,* 120–129.

McFarlane, J. M., Groff, J. Y., O'Brien, J. A., & Watson, K. (2005). Behaviors of children exposed to intimate partner violence before and 1 year after a treatment program for their mother. *Applied Nursing Research, 18,* 7–12.

Merry, S. N., Stasiak, K., Shepherd, M., Frampton, C., Fleming, T., & Lucassen, M. F. (2012). The effectiveness of SPARX, a computerised self help intervention for adolescents seeking help for depression: Randomised controlled non-inferiority trial. *British Medical Journal, 344,* e2598.

Midgley, N., & Kennedy, E. (2011). Psychodynamic psychotherapy for children and adolescents: A critical review of the evidence base. *Journal of Child Psychotherapy, 37,* 232–260.

Miklowitz, D. J., Biuckians, A., & Richards, J. A. (2006). Early-onset bipolar disorder: A family treatment perspective. *Development and Psychopathology, 18,* 1247–1265.

Moss, E., Dubois-Comtois, K., Cyr, C., Tarabulsy, G. M., St-Laurent, D., & Bernier, A. (2011). Efficacy of a home-visiting intervention aimed at improving maternal sensitivity, child attachment, and behavioral outcomes for maltreated children: A randomized control trial. *Development and Psychopathology, 23,* 195–210.

Munoz-Solomando, A., Kendall, T., & Whittington, C. J. (2008). Cognitive behavioural therapy for children and adolescents. *Current Opinion in Psychiatry, 21,* 332–337.

Muratori, F., Picchi, L., Bruni, G., Patarnello, M., & Romagnoli, G. (2003). A two-year follow-up of psychodynamic psychotherapy for internalizing disorders in children. *Journal of the American Academy of Child and Adolescent Psychiatry, 42,* 331–339.

National Institute for Health and Clinical Excellence. (2005). Depression in children and young people: Identification and management in primary, community and secondary care. Clinical Guideline CG28. London: National Institute for Health and Clinical Excellence.

National Institute for Health and Clinical Excellence. (2009). Antisocial personality disorder: Treatment, management and prevention. London: National Institute for Health and Clinical Excellence.

National Institute for Health and Clinical Excellence. (2013). *Conduct disorders and antisocial behaviour in children and young people: Recognition, intervention and management (CG158).* London: British Psychological Society and Royal College of Psychiatrists.

Office of Program Policy Analysis & Government Accountability. (2007). Redirection pilots meet and exceed residential commitment outcomes; $5.8 million saved. Tallahassee, FL: Florida Legislature.

Ozonoff, S., & Miller, J. N. (1995). Teaching theory of mind: A new approach to social skills training for individuals with autism. *Journal of Autism and Developmental Disorders, 25,* 415–433.

Pavuluri, M. N., Graczyk, P. A., Henry, D. B., Carbray, J. A., Heidenreich, J., & Miklowitz, D. J. (2004). Child- and family-focused cognitive-behavioral therapy for pediatric bipolar disorder: Development and preliminary results. *Journal of the American Academy of Child and Adolescent Psychiatry, 43,* 528–537.

Peters-Scheffer, N., Didden, R., Korzilius, H., & Sturmey, P. (2011). A meta-analytic study on the effectiveness of comprehensive ABA-based early intervention programs for children with autism spectrum disorders. *Research in Autism Spectrum Disorders, 5,* 60–69.

Petrosino, A., Turpin-Petrosino, C., & Guckenburg, S. (2010). Formal system processing of juveniles: Effects on delinquency. *Campbell Systematic Reviews 2010,* 1.

Pfiffner, L. J., Yee Mikami, A., Huang-Pollock, C., Easterlin, B., Zalecki, C., & McBurnett, K. (2007). A randomized, controlled trial of integrated home-school behavioral treatment for ADHD, predominantly inattentive type. *Journal of the American Academy of Child and Adolescent Psychiatry, 46,* 1041–1050.

Piacentini, J., Bergman, R. L., Chang, S., Langley, A., Peris, T., Wood, J. J., et al. (2011). Controlled comparison of family cognitive behavioral therapy and psychoeducation/relaxation training for child obsessive-compulsive disorder. *Journal of the American Academy of Child and Adolescent Psychiatry, 50,* 1149–1161.

Pilling, S., Bebbington, P., Kuipers, E., Garety, P., Geddes, J., Martindale, B., . . . Morgan, C. (2002). Psychological treatments in schizophrenia: II. Meta-analyses of randomized controlled trials of social skills training and cognitive remediation. *Psychological Medicine, 32,* 783–791.

Pliszka, S., & AACAP Work Group on Quality Issues. (2007). Practice parameter for the assessment and treatment of children and adolescents with attention-deficit/hyperactivity disorder. *Journal of the American Academy of Child and Adolescent Psychiatry, 46,* 894–921.

Rathus, J. H., & Miller, A. L. (2002). Dialectical behavior therapy adapted for suicidal adolescents. *Suicide and Life-Threatening Behavior, 32,* 146–157.

Redondo, S., Garrido, V., & Sánchez-Meca, J. (1997). What works in correctional rehabilitation in Europe: A meta-analytic review. In S. Redondo, V. Garrido, J. Pérez & R. Barberet (Eds.), *Advances in psychology and law: International contributions* (pp. 499–523). Berlin: De Gruyter.

Reeker, J., Ensing, D., & Elliott, R. (1997). A meta-analytic investigation of group treatment outcomes for sexually abused children. *Child Abuse & Neglect, 21,* 669–680.

Reyno, S. M., & McGrath, P. J. (2006). Predictors of parent training efficacy for child externalizing behavior problems – a meta-analytic review. *Journal of Child Psychology and Psychiatry, 47,* 99–111.

Rosselló, J., & Bernal, G. (1999). The efficacy of cognitive-behavioral and interpersonal treatments for depression in Puerto Rican adolescents. *Journal of Consulting and Clinical Psychology, 67,* 734–745.

Rosselló, J., Bernal, G., & Rivera-Medina, C. (2008). Individual and group CBT and IPT for Puerto Rican adolescents with depressive symptoms. *Cultural Diversity and Ethnic Minority Psychology*, 14, 234–245.

Roth, A., & Fonagy, P. (2005). *What works for whom? A critical review of psychotherapy research* (2nd ed.). New York: Guilford Press.

Rund, B. R., Moe, L., Sollien, T., Fjell, A., Borchgrevink, T., Hallert, M., & Naess, P. O. (1994). The Psychosis Project: Outcome and cost-effectiveness of a psychoeducational treatment program for schizophrenic adolescents. *Acta Psychiatrica Scandinavica*, 89, 211–218.

Saavedra, L. M., Silverman, W. K., Morgan-Lopez, A. A., & Kurtines, W. M. (2010). Cognitive behavioral treatment for childhood anxiety disorders: Long-term effects on anxiety and secondary disorders in young adulthood. *Journal of Child Psychology and Psychiatry*, 51, 924–934.

Sackett, D. L., Rosenberg, W. M. C., Gray, J. A. M., Haynes, R. B., & Richardson, W. S. (1996). Evidence based medicine: What it is and what it isn't. *British Medical Journal*, 312, 71–72.

Safran, J. D., Muran, J. C., & Eubanks-Carter, C. (2011). Repairing alliance ruptures. *Psychotherapy*, 48, 80–87.

Sánchez-Meca, J., Rosa-Alcázar, A. I., & López-Soler, C. (2011). The psychological treatment of sexual abuse in children and adolescents: A meta-analysis. *International Journal of Clinical and Health Psychology*, 11, 67–93.

Santisteban, D. A., Coatsworth, J. D., Perez-Vidal, A., Kurtines, W. M., Schwartz, S. J., LaPerriere, A., & Szapocznik, J. (2003). Efficacy of brief strategic family therapy in modifying Hispanic adolescent behavior problems and substance use. *Journal of Family Psychology*, 17, 121–133.

Scahill, L., Aman, M. G., McDougle, C. J., McCracken, J. T., Tierney, E., Dziura, J., . . . Vitiello, B. (2006). A prospective open trial of guanfacine in children with pervasive developmental disorders. *Journal of Child and Adolescent Psychopharmacology*, 16, 589–598.

Schaal, S., Elbert, T., & Neuner, F. (2009). Narrative exposure therapy versus interpersonal psychotherapy: A pilot randomized controlled trial with Rwandan genocide orphans. *Psychotherapy and Psychosomatics*, 78, 298–306.

Scheeringa, M. S., Weems, C. F., Cohen, J. A., Amaya-Jackson, L., & Guthrie, D. (2011). Trauma-focused cognitive-behavioral therapy for posttraumatic stress disorder in three-through six-year-old children: A randomized clinical trial. *Journal of Child Psychology and Psychiatry*, 52, 853–860.

Schmidt, U., Lee, S., Beecham, J., Perkins, S., Treasure, J., Yi, I., . . . Eisler, I. (2007). A randomized controlled trial of family therapy and cognitive behavior therapy guided self-care for adolescents with bulimia nervosa and related disorders. *American Journal of Psychiatry*, 164, 591–598.

Scott, S., Sylva, K., Doolan, M., Price, J., Jacobs, B., Crook, C., & Landau, S. (2010). Randomised controlled trial of parent groups for child antisocial behaviour targeting multiple risk factors: The SPOKES project. *Journal of Child Psychology and Psychiatry*, 51, 48–57.

Seligman, M. E. P. (1996). Science as an ally of practice. *American Psychologist*, 51, 1072–1079.

Sexton, T., & Turner, C. W. (2010). The effectiveness of functional family therapy for youth with behavioral problems in a community practice setting. *Journal of Family Psychology*, 24, 339–348.

Silverman, W. K., Kurtines, W. M., Ginsburg, G. S., Weems, C. F., Lumpkin, P. W., & Carmichael, D. H. (1999). Treating anxiety disorders in children with group cognitive-behavioral therapy: A randomized clinical trial. *Journal of Consulting and Clinical Psychology*, 67, 995–1003.

Sofronoff, K., Attwood, T., & Hinton, S. (2005). A randomised controlled trial of a CBT intervention for anxiety in children with Asperger syndrome. *Journal of Child Psychology and Psychiatry*, 46, 1152–1160.

Sofronoff, K., Leslie, A., & Brown, W. (2004). Parent management training and Asperger syndrome: A randomized controlled trial to evaluate a parent based intervention. *Autism*, 8, 301–317.

Solomon, M., Goodlin-Jones, B. L., & Anders, T. F. (2004). A social adjustment enhancement intervention for high functioning autism, Asperger's syndrome, and pervasive developmental disorder NOS. *Journal of Autism and Developmental Disorders*, 34, 649–668.

Southam-Gerow, M. A., Kendall, P. C., & Weersing, V. R. (2001). Examining outcome variability: Correlates of treatment response in a child and adolescent anxiety clinic. *Journal of Clinical Child Psychology*, 30, 422–436.

Southam-Gerow, M. A., Weisz, J. R., Chu, B. C., McLeod, B. D., Gordis, E. B., & Connor-Smith, J. K. (2011). Does cognitive behavioral therapy for youth anxiety outperform usual care in community clinics? An initial effectiveness test. *Journal of the American Academy of Child and Adolescent Psychiatry*, 49, 1043–1052.

Spence, S. H., Donovan, C. L., March, S., Gamble, A., Anderson, R. E., Prosser, S., & Kenardy, J. (2011). A randomized controlled trial of online versus clinic-based CBT for adolescent anxiety. *Journal of Consulting and Clinical Psychology*, 79, 629–642.

Spielmans, G. I., Pasek, L. F., & McFall, J. P. (2007). What are the active ingredients in cognitive and behavioral psychotherapy for anxious and depressed children? A meta-analytic review. *Clinical Psychology Review*, 27, 642–654.

Spring, B. (2007). Evidence-based practice in clinical psychology: What it is, why it matters; what you need to know. *Journal of Clinical Psychology*, 63, 611–631.

Stark, K. D., Hargrave, J., Hersh, B., Greenberg, M., Herren, J., & Fisher, M. (2008). Treatment of childhood depression: The ACTION program. In J. R. Z. Abela & B. L. Hankin (Eds.), *Handbook of depression in children and adolescents* (pp. 224–249). New York: Guilford Press.

Stein, B. D., Jaycox, L. H., Kataoka, S. H., Wong, M., Tu, W., Elliott, M. N., & Fink, A. (2003). A mental health intervention for schoolchildren exposed to violence: A randomized controlled trial. *Journal of the American Medical Association*, 290, 603–611.

Storch, E. A., Lehmkuhl, H. D., Ricketts, E., Geffken, G. R., Marien, W., & Murphy, T. K. (2010). An open trial of intensive family based cognitive-behavioral therapy in youth with obsessive-compulsive disorder who are medication partial responders or nonresponders. *Journal of Clinical Child and Adolescent Psychology*, 39, 260–268.

Sukhodolsky, D. G., Kassinove, H., & Gorman, B. S. (2004). Cognitive-behavioral therapy for anger in children and adolescents: A meta-analysis. *Aggression and Violent Behavior*, 9, 247–269.

Suter, J., & Bruns, E. J. (2008). A narrative review of wraparound outcome studies. In E. J. Bruns & J. S. Walker (Eds.), *The resource guide to wraparound*. Portland, OR: National Wraparound Initiative, Research and Training Center for Family Support and Children's Mental Health.

Suter, J. C., & Bruns, E. J. (2009). Effectiveness of the wraparound process for children with emotional and behavioral disorders: A meta-analysis. *Clinical Child and Family Psychology Review*, 12, 336–351.

Swenson, C. C., Schaeffer, C. M., Henggeler, S. W., Faldowski, R., & Mayhew, A. M. (2010). Multisystemic therapy for child abuse and neglect: A randomized effectiveness trial. *Journal of Family Psychology*, 24, 497–507.

Taussig, H. N., Clyman, R. B., & Landsverk, J. (2001). Children who return home from foster care: A 6-year prospective study of behavioral health outcomes in adolescence. *Pediatrics*, 108, E10.

Toth, S. L., Maughan, A., Manly, J. T., Spagnola, M., & Cicchetti, D. (2002). The relative efficacy of two interventions in altering maltreated preschool children's representational models: Implications for attachment theory. *Development and Psychopathology*, 14, 877–908.

Trask, E. V., Walsh, K., & Dilillo, D. (2011). Treatment effects for common outcomes of child sexual abuse: A current meta-analysis. *Aggression and Violent Behavior*, 16, 6–19.

Trowell, J., Joffe, I., Campbell, J., Clemente, C., Almqvist, F., Soininen, M., . . . Tsiantis, J. (2007). Childhood depression: A place for psychotherapy. An outcome study comparing individual psychodynamic psychotherapy and family therapy. *European Child & Adolescent Psychiatry*, 16, 157–167.

Trowell, J., Kolvin, I., Weeramanthri, T., Sadowski, H., Berelowitz, M., Glaser, D., & Leitch, I. (2002). Psychotherapy for sexually abused girls: Psychopathological outcome findings and patterns of change. *British Journal of Psychiatry*, 180, 234–247.

Udwin, O. (1983). Imaginative play training as an intervention method with institutionalised preschool children. *British Journal of Educational Psychology*, 53(Pt 1), 32–39.

Vostanis, P., Feehan, C., Grattan, E., & Bickerton, W. L. (1996). A randomised controlled out-patient trial of cognitive-behavioural treatment for children and adolescents with depression: 9-month follow-up. *Journal of Affective Disorders*, 40, 105–116.

Waldron, H. B., Slesnick, N., Brody, J. L., Turner, C. W., & Peterson, T. R. (2001). Treatment outcomes for adolescent substance abuse at 4- and 7-month assessments. *Journal of Consulting and Clinical Psychology*, 69, 802–813.

Walker, H. M., Colvin, G., & Ramsey, E. (1995). *Antisocial behavior in school: Strategies and best practices*. Pacific Grove, CA: Brooks/Cole.

Wampold, B. E. (1997). Methodological problems in identifying efficacious psychotherapies. *Psychotherapy Research*, 7, 21–43.

Waters, A. M., Ford, L. A., Wharton, T. A., & Cobham, V. E. (2009). Cognitive-behavioural therapy for young children with anxiety disorders: Comparison of a child + parent condition versus a parent only condition. *Behaviour Research and Therapy*, 47, 654–662.

Webster-Stratton, C., & Reid, M. J. (2010). The Incredible Years parents, teachers and children training series: A multifaceted treatment approach for young children with conduct disorders. In A. E. Kazdin & J. R. Weisz (Eds.), *Evidence-based psychotherapies for children and adolescents* (2nd ed.) (pp. 194–210). New York: Guilford Press.

Weisz, J. R., Chorpita, B. F., Palinkas, L. A., Schoenwald, S. K., Miranda, J., Bearman, S. K., . . . Research Network on Youth Mental Health. (2012). Testing standard and modular designs for psychotherapy treating depression, anxiety, and conduct problems in youth: A randomized effectiveness trial. *Archives of General Psychiatry*, 69, 274–282.

Weisz, J. R., Doss, A. J., & Hawley, K. (2005). Youth psychotherapy outcome research: A review and critique of the evidence base. *Annual Review of Psychology*, 56, 337–363.

Weisz, J. R., Jensen-Doss, A., & Hawley, K. M. (2006). Evidence-based youth psychotherapies versus usual clinical care: A meta-analysis of direct comparisons. *American Psychologist*, 61, 671–689.

Westermark, P. K., Hansson, K., & Olsson, M. (2011). Multidimensional treatment foster care (MTFC): Results from an independent replication. *Journal of Family Therapy*, 33, 20–41.

Wethington, H. R., Hahn, R. A., Fuqua-Whitley, D. S., Sipe, T. A., Crosby, A. E., Johnson, R. L., . . . Task Force on Community Preventive Services. (2008). The effectiveness of interventions to reduce psychological harm from traumatic events among children and adolescents: A systematic review. *American Journal of Preventive Medicine*, 35, 287–313.

Williams, T. I., Salkovskis, P. M., Forrester, L., Turner, S., White, H., & Allsopp, M. A. (2010). A randomised controlled trial of cognitive behavioural treatment for obsessive compulsive disorder in children and adolescents. *European Child & Adolescent Psychiatry*, 19, 449–456.

Wilson, S. J., & Lipsey, M. W. (2007). School-based interventions for aggressive and disruptive behavior: Update of a meta-analysis. *American Journal of Preventive Medicine*, 33(Suppl. 2), S130–143.

Zeanah, C. H., Larrieu, J. A., Heller, S. S., Valliere, J., Hinshaw-Fuselier, S., Aoki, Y., & Drilling, M. (2001). Evaluation of a preventive intervention for maltreated infants and toddlers in foster care. *Journal of the American Academy of Child and Adolescent Psychiatry*, 40, 214–221.

6

WHAT LEADS TO CHANGE? I. COMMON FACTORS IN CHILD THERAPY

JACQUELINE HAYES

This chapter discusses

This chapter discusses the evidence for different factors that contribute to therapeutic change in children and young people, including:

- The impact of the therapy relationship and therapeutic alliance
- The role of children and young people in their own change
- What therapists can do to increase the likelihood of a child or young person engaging with and benefiting from therapy
- The role of parents and caregivers in successful therapy
- Whether or not the setting in which therapy takes place influences how much children and young people benefit from therapy
- The gaps in the research evidence in these areas and ideas for future enquiry

Please note that this chapter will use the term 'caregiver' to refer to those who have responsibility for looking after a child or young person – including biological parents, and also legal guardians. The term 'parent/s' will be used where a specific research study/paper itself has talked about parents.

Introduction

What are common factors?

In adult therapies, researchers for many years now have tried to isolate, and measure the various 'active ingredients' of psychotherapies (see Cooper, 2008). This is not merely an academic concern because if we can work out which features of therapy are most important in bringing about change, this gives us a chance to design services that will maximize the potential for engagement from clients in the process, and potentially enhance the potency of our work. However, it is also worth being clear about the limits of empirical research – it is often based on averages and, even when a research finding is true for people *in general*, that does not necessarily mean it is true for the particular child or young person you are working with.

Really what we are speaking of when we talk about any evidence in therapy is *the probability, or the likelihood, that some feature of a client, attribute of a therapist or therapeutic process, will lead to more therapeutic change, as based on a measure that approximates therapeutic change.* As discussed in the introduction to this book, empirical evidence forms an important source of information from which to work, which may challenge our theoretical, personal or societal assumptions in a way that is healthy and enhances our capacity for growth.

Common factors is a phrase used in psychotherapy research that refers to those active ingredients that are not associated with just one, or a collection of schools of therapy – examples of the modality-specific factors might be 'congruence' in person-centred therapy or 'transference' in psychodynamic therapy. What we instead refer to is those features that could, in theory (and practice), be found in any type of psychotherapy. In adults, such common factors are now thought to be possibly the most important contributors to therapeutic change (Cooper, 2008), with 'client factors' – such as their motivation to change – among the most vital.

In child and adolescent therapy, just as the clients are younger, so too is the research. Few of the potential factors identified in adult research, apart from the 'therapeutic alliance' which we will examine shortly, have been studied across a range of therapies and with a wide variety of children and young people. Thus, many of the findings reported here should be treated as tentative initial indications rather than trends and patterns that we can be fairly sure of. Having said that, we can of course consider these findings in the context of what we know from other sources of information – such as the findings from adult therapy, the conceptual models that guide our work, or the 'findings' from our own experiences as therapists and clients.

The therapy relationship

> The first condition specifies that a minimal relationship, a psychological contact, must exist. I am hypothesizing that significant positive personality change does not occur except in a relationship. This is of course a hypothesis, and it may be disproved. (Rogers, 1957: 96)

However we define it, most schools of therapy acknowledge the fact that psychotherapy takes place within the context of an interpersonal relationship. This chapter follows Proctor (2014) in using the term 'therapy relationship' rather than 'therapeutic relationship', as this does not assume that it is inevitably therapeutic.

There are divergences between different models of therapy on how and why the therapy relationship is important to understand; for example, in the humanistic tradition, the therapeutic relationship is considered the vehicle for change – providing the conditions in which growth can occur. In the cognitive and behavioural traditions, the alliance is believed to be the means through which the work of therapy can be made possible; the way coop-eration between therapist and client can be established and thus, essential for the other agents of change – tasks and techniques – to take place.

In adult therapies, the therapy relationship is strongly associated with successful therapeutic work – overlapping about 30 per cent with treatment outcomes (see Asay & Lambert, 1999). Could it be that in child and adolescent therapy – where children often have not chosen to access therapy, and where others may even be more distressed by their problems than they are (Shirk & Saiz, 1992) – forming a good relationship with a therapist becomes even more important?

Researchers have broken the therapy relationship down into various parts (Karver, Handelsman, Fields, & Bickman, 2006) and these include the following:

- Therapeutic alliance (discussed below)
- Affect towards the therapist (discussed below)
- The autonomy the client shows in therapy (see 'client factors', below)
- The client's willingness to participate (see 'client factors', below)
- The therapist's style of interpersonal relating (see 'therapist factors', below)
- Therapist self-disclosure (see Chapter 7 on therapeutic attitudes and techniques).

Karver et al. (2006) estimate that 'therapeutic relationship variables' have an **effect size** of 0.54 (d) on outcomes in child therapy. This is a medium effect in Cohen's terms, and includes all of these individual components. The most researched therapy relationship factor, however, is something called the 'therapeutic alliance'. It is this we turn to first.

The therapeutic alliance

The alliance between the child and therapist was first spoken of by Anna Freud (1946). She emphasized the importance of an emotional connection between the two as under-pinning all the other work of therapy. This separation between emotional connection, or bond, in therapy, and the tasks of therapy, has been formative for the literature in this area and structures most of the research that has come since. Although early empirical measures of the therapeutic alliance were largely shaped by psychodynamic thinking, more recent work, including the widely used Working Alliance Inventory (Horvath & Greenberg, 1989), is more influenced by cognitive behavioural ideas. In fact, contemporary research in this area tends to follow Bordin's (1979) definition of alliance as being made up of three components: (1) emotional bond, (2) task collabora-tion and (3) agreements on goals. Box 6.1 below summarizes some research issues involved in measuring the alliance.

How does the child–therapist alliance relate to measured outcomes?

Several recent **meta-analyses** indicate that the **correlation** between the therapeutic alliance with the child or young person, and outcomes is in the range of $r = 0.14$ to 0.22 (Karver et al., 2006; McLeod, 2011; Shirk & Karver, 2003; Shirk et al., 2011).

This is a Cohen's d of between 0.28 and 0.45 and is thus a small to medium effect. Shirk and Karver (2011) conclude that based on these estimates the alliance explains about 4 per cent of the overall **variance** in therapeutic outcomes (using the figure of 0.2). This is equivalent to estimates of the contribution that specific techniques make to successful therapy (see Miller, Wampold, & Varhely, 2008; more on this in Chapter 7).

Furthermore, this contribution to outcomes is just as important in behavioural therapies and non-behavioural therapies, 'in treatments as different as manual-guided CBT and non-directive play therapy' (Shirk & Karver, 2011: 82). The relationship between alliance and outcomes appears to be strongest with children (under 12) as opposed to adolescents (r = 0.27 and 0.17 respectively; Shirk & Karver, 2011). One study has specifically focused on the first aspect of Bordin's therapeutic alliance – the child's bond with the therapist – and found a small to moderate relationship between a positive bond and good therapeutic outcomes (Berg, 1999, as cited in Karver et al., 2006). (This section is about the child/young person's alliance with their therapist, but there is also the issue of the caregiver–therapist working relationship, which will be considered below.)

Some researchers have checked what the direction of the relationship is between strong alliances and good outcomes. For example, does a strong alliance early in the therapeutic process lead to more benefits for children and young people – or, does it work in the other direction, that improvements early in therapy lead children and young people to see the alliance as stronger or better in some way, which in turn leads to better outcomes by the end of therapy? A study of young people diagnosed with depression tested these two different **hypotheses** and found most support for the idea that a strong alliance early in therapy drives more therapeutic change, rather than the other way round (Labouliere, Reyes, Shirk, & Karver, 2015). The same researchers also found that the severity of depression experienced by young people did not predict the strength of their alliance with their therapist – in other words, being very depressed did not prevent them from forming strong working alliances with their therapists (Labouliere et al., 2015).

Box 6.1   How is the alliance measured?

The answer to this question is – in many ways! Shirk et al. (2011) in their meta-analysis identified 10 different measures in just 16 studies. They found the two most commonly used questionnaires to be the Working Alliance Inventory (WAI) and the Therapeutic Alliance Scale for Children (TASC). Examples of items from the WAI include:

- 'My therapist and I understood each other'
- 'I disagreed with my therapist on what I wanted to get out of therapy'
- 'I was worried about the outcome of the sessions'

These are rated on a seven-point scale from 'never' to 'always' (Horvath & Greenberg, 1989). The WAI tends to be used more with young people while the TASC is used more with children (Shirk et al., 2011). The alliance is also investigated using qualitative methods, which are important for capturing variety and depth of responses, and an example of such a study appears below in Box 6.3.

Another important question is who should be rating the alliance? Should it be the child or young person, the therapist, the caregivers, independent observers, or all of the above? One paper highlighted just how differently the alliance can look from these perspectives, finding that, firstly, parent views of the alliance were much more strongly related to outcomes than their child's reports. Secondly, there was a lot less **variance** or difference between different children's ratings of the alliance than between different parents', with children rating alliances with their therapist more homogeneously as positive (McLeod, 2011).

A further complication concerns when in therapy to assess alliance. Most of the research reported here is based on studies that assess the alliance early in therapy. Should it also be measured at the end of therapy, or periodically during the process? One meta-analysis found that there were weaker associations between alliance and outcomes when alliance was measured earlier, as opposed to later, in the process – but which measurement do we trust as 'closer to the truth'? Does this suggest that later measurements might be less reliable due to being **confounded** with improvements in symptoms, as the author suggested (McLeod, 2011), or might the later measurements be more valid because it simply takes some time to establish alliances and rate them fairly? And if we measure the alliance at different points in the process, how might the very act of measurement itself affect the alliance?

What does the research say about strengthening the alliance?

Given that forming a strong working alliance is associated with better outcomes for children and young people, several studies have tried to investigate what elements are involved when an alliance is strong or weak. Most of these studies have been run by researchers in the cognitive behavioural tradition, and Box 6.2 summarizes the results from several of these.

Box 6.2   Research on strong and weak alliance

Factors associated with weak alliances:

- Failure to respond to the child's expressions of emotion
- Pushing children to talk
- A strong emphasis on discussing problems
- Speaking to the child in a very formal way
- Being overfamiliar and overemphasizing 'common-ground' – for example, therapist saying 'I like that music too!' in a false or forced manner

Factors associated with strong alliances:

- Pace of therapy is set by the child
- Goals of therapy are set by the child
- Therapist presents therapy as a team effort
- The therapist is mindful of the child's level of tolerance in discussing emotionally difficult topics

Chu and Kendall (2009), Creed and Kendall (2005), Jungbluth and Shirk (2009).

One study in this area, by Jungbluth and Shirk (2009), investigated first sessions of therapy with adolescents who were receiving CBT for a diagnosis of depression. They found that therapists who imposed less structure in the initial session were more likely to have adolescents who showed greater participation in their therapy subsequently. 'Less structure' in this case meant providing space for greater exploration of the adolescents' experiences and stories. In their review of the area, Shirk and Karver (2011: 87) conclude that the initial findings from five CBT studies suggest that 'a less directive and task focused approach to therapy is critical at the start of treatment. Efforts to engage the client by pushing or praising are contraindicated . . . and suggest that client-centred strategies at the start of therapy may be more effective for alliance formation.'

Research from the humanistic field also supports such an approach, as Box 6.3 details.

Box 6.3   Key studies: What helps adolescents to express themselves in therapy?

Sagen, Hummelsund and Binder (2013) asked young people about the relational factors that helped them to express themselves in therapy. They found five themes that their informants' responses clustered around:

- Theme 1: receiving full and genuine attention
- Theme 2: being accepted and valued
- Theme 3: the therapist staying with them through emotionally painful moments
- Theme 4: not having to take responsibility for their therapist's wellbeing
- Theme 5: the therapist facilitating openness through sharing. Some adolescents really valued their therapist sharing something about themselves, helping them to open up about themselves too. However, others preferred not to know too much so that they did not feel responsible for their therapist (see Chapter 7 for more on self-disclosure).

Some adolescents demonstrated these helpful aspects by contrasting how their therapist compared to other adults in their lives; for example one young person said:

'My father often says, "that is no problem, just do it". My therapist is not like that, she lets me complain. That is a good feeling, to be able to do that without being told, "Oh my God, you are so stupid". She does not judge me for it – she is not annoyed at me complaining. She listens to me complaining, and that feels good.' (Sagen et al., 2013: 66–67)

Box 6.4   Implications for practice

Together, these initial results suggest that being a genuinely *responsive, flexible* and caring adult, *rather than trying to be similar* to the child or young person, is most important in allowing them to trust and form a good relationship with their therapist. These studies also emphasize the importance, particularly at the start of therapy, of children and young people influencing the topics and pacing, even in more pre-structured or technique-based therapies.

Child factors

So far, we have seen that a therapeutic relationship with a therapist is an important factor associated with change in therapy. However, a small to medium effect size suggests that it does not account for all change – there must be many other ingredients that are contributing to therapeutic change that are not necessarily about the therapy relationship. One of these might be the characteristics that children and young people bring that influence how much benefit they receive from therapy.

In child and adolescent therapy there has been a comparatively small amount of research looking at what characteristics of children and their caregivers are associated with good outcomes. These might be demographic factors such as age, ethnicity or gender; or issues related more to their motivations and perceptions. What these things have in common is that they are all features that researchers have attempted to measure, or ask children and young people directly about, and that they have a particular focus on the person as an individual rather than the therapist or the therapy itself. In adult therapy, client factors such as levels of social support, or tendencies towards thinking psychologically before therapy, are estimated to be the biggest contributors to change in therapy (Cooper, 2008). In child and adolescent therapy, a child's characteristics have been linked to two different types of 'outcomes': (1) end-of-therapy outcomes – how much change in the child/adolescent has been observed by the end of therapy; and (2) within-therapy outcomes – the impact on the formation of a therapeutic alliance. (Later in the chapter we will look at caregiver factors in more detail.)

Expectations of therapy

There is a small amount of research looking at the link between expectations and outcome in young people. These studies have explored if children and young people know what to expect from therapy; and whether or not any expectations they might have link to outcomes. Both areas have recently been investigated both qualitatively and quantitatively. In one study, the researchers interviewed 20 young people immediately prior to the first therapy session. They found a prevailing theme that most young people were simply unsure of what to expect and, interestingly, this was even despite the fact that most of them had received therapy previously. The study concluded that 'the young people did not know what to expect with regard to their role as a client, who they would see, and what the person would be like, or the format of the sessions' (Watsford, Rickwood, & Vanags, 2013: 135). Another study, featured in Box 6.5, investigated the same topic, finding some similar themes but also some new ones, including that some young people did in fact have clear expectations of what their therapist might be like. Much less is known about the expectations of younger children, although some studies (e.g. Carlberg, Thorén, Billström, & Odhammar, 2009), have explored this.

So how much do expectations matter, in terms of outcomes? We cannot be sure of exactly what influence this has, because there is so little to go on in this area. In one survey of 228 young people aged 12–25 years, Watsford and Rickwood (2014) found no link between their initial expectations and how well they did in therapy. This needs testing in further studies but, if this pattern holds up, it is contrary to the pattern observed in studies with adults (see Cooper, 2008). However, as we shall see below, parental expectations of therapy may be more influential.

Box 6.5   Key studies: Hopes and expectations for therapy in depressed adolescents

One study has examined the expectations for therapy of 77 young people, aged 11–17, referred to child and adolescent mental health services (CAMHS), who were diagnosed with moderate to severe depression. The authors stated their aims as wanting to 'investigate the ideas that young people have going into therapy, a sense of the otherwise unspoken feelings of young people, and thus help clinicians negotiate the delicate early phases of treatment' (Midgley, Holmes, Parkinson, Stapley, Eatough, & Target, 2016: 13). They used **semi-structured interviews**, and their analysis yielded the following themes:

- **'I dunno': The difficulty of imagining what will happen in therapy.** The authors described this lack of expectation as the most 'persistently striking feature of these interviews' (Midgley et al., 2016: 15), which reinforces Watsford et al.'s (2013) findings detailed above. However Midgley et al. (2016) also observed that this phrase was used in different ways by the young people – sometimes to express a desperation and exasperation with their problems, at other times to express a reluctance to engage, or also showing an unwillingness or embarrassment to go into detail with the interviewer.
- **The 'talking cure'.** The majority of young people had an expectation that therapy would involve doing some talking, although they differed in what they imagined this talking would involve. Some imagined the therapist would be more like a doctor – 'They talk to you and give you a bit of medicine'. The therapist was seen as a medical expert who asks questions and finds clues to establish where their problems had come from, before recommending a course of treatment to cure the problem. However, others imagined therapy as more of a relationship – some young people imagined a less hierarchical situation, where they would need to build up a relationship with the therapist over time, and that person would help them to find ways to solve their own problems. For a comparable study describing the expectations of depressed adolescents in Germany, see Weitkamp, Klein, & Midgley (2016).

Box 6.6   Implications for practice

The findings from qualitative research point to the fact that many adolescents may not know what to expect from therapy, or have rather specific ideas about what a therapist is going to be like, sometimes based on media images of 'the shrink'. Given this, therapists working with young people need to be mindful that the expectations that young people have for their therapy may not align with their own. It could be useful to explore what those expectations are, and to explain to young people, when starting therapy, the kinds of things that happen in sessions and the ways in which therapy differs from going to see a doctor about medical problems.

Readiness for change

One important difference between child and adult therapies is that in the case of children, especially younger ones, they are much less likely to have referred themselves to therapy, and often may be unsure as to why they are there and quite what to expect from the interaction. We therefore might expect there may be less 'readiness to change'. But does the research suggest that this matters?

Research in child and adolescent therapy mostly corroborates findings in the adult field, namely that those who see themselves as having a problem, who have reasons for wanting to change their actions, and who therefore have greater motivation to participate in therapy, form better alliances with their therapist (Estrada & Russell, 1999; Fitzpatrick & Irannejad, 2008). For example, one study found that young people who had greater motivation to abstain from drugs, had better therapeutic outcomes in terms of less substance use by the end of therapy (Black & Chung, 2014). This is a similar idea to 'motivation to change'. Similarly, 'commitment to therapy' was measured by Adelman, Kaser-Boyd and Taylor (1984). They found that those young people who showed more commitment to therapy had better overall therapeutic outcomes. However, the picture is again more complex, as Killips, Cooper, Freire and McGinnis (2012) found in their sample of young people receiving school-based counselling that 'client motivation' was not associated with outcomes.

Involvement

The degree to which children and young people are involved in their therapy, and willing to be involved, does seem to be associated with how much benefit they get from therapy. A meta-analysis found that a child or young person's 'willingness to participate' and 'actual participation' in therapy were associated with outcomes (Karver et al., 2006). The authors estimated the effect size of both features to be $d = 0.56$ – in other words, a medium effect size.

A recent survey study found that those young people that showed 'a preference for being personally committed to therapy', before the start of therapy, experienced more change by the end of therapy (Watsford & Rickwood, 2014). The higher they rated their preference to be personally committed to therapy, before therapy started, the more likely they would be to enjoy improved psychological functioning by the end of therapy. Gorin and Gorin (1993) took the same topic and measured this from a slightly different angle. This study used observers to rate the behaviour of children and parents on admission to a service, and also therapists' ratings of how the process of therapy unfolded. They found, similarly, that levels of client engagement in therapy were the most important predictor of therapeutic outcomes, and mattered much more than factors such as **demographic variables** (including age and diagnosis), or treatment methods.

Some studies have also measured what has been termed 'client autonomy' – a 'demonstration of self-direction in his/her relationship with a therapist' (Karver et al., 2006: 53). A meta-analysis of studies involving children and young people found this to be **correlated** with outcomes, though this had a smaller effect ($d = 0.3$).

Although based on a relatively small number of studies, taken together this research suggests that:

- children and young people who want to change are more likely to engage with a therapist once therapy begins;
- those who show greater involvement in therapy get more out of therapy;
- those who show more autonomy with their therapist are more likely to benefit from the therapeutic encounter.

Age of child/adolescent

The findings are inconclusive as to whether younger or older children benefit most from psychotherapy. For example, Bratton, Ray, Rhine and Jones's (2005) meta-analysis of play therapy and Kendall, Hudson, Gosch, Flannery-Schroeder and Suveg's (2009) study of CBT (as cited in McLaughlin, Holliday, Clarke, & Ilie, 2013) found that a client's age did not influence how effective therapy was. Similarly, another study found that these factors did not seem to influence how much clients benefited in therapies for depression and anxiety (Nilsen, Eisemann, & Kvernmo, 2013). However, other studies have found age to be important. A recent meta-analysis of play therapies by Lin and Bratton (2015) indicated that children less than 8 years old benefited more from play therapy. Similarly, a study of cases of child and adolescent psychoanalysis showed that children (less than 12 years) benefited more from their intensive therapies than adolescents (Target & Fonagy, 1994). However, when it comes to school-based therapy, adolescents have been found to benefit more than children (Baskin, Slaten, Crosby, Pufahl, Schneller, & Ladell, 2010). The effect of age on outcomes is thus inconclusive and it is probably likely that any differential effects will be found in specific types of therapy that may suit older, or younger children.

Gender and ethnicity

Preliminary evidence suggests that the gender of a child or adolescent receiving therapy does not seem to make a difference to therapeutic outcomes. Boys and girls seem to derive the same amount of benefit from therapy, in the largest studies that have tested this (Bratton et al., 2005; Nilsen et al., 2013).

When it comes to ethnicity, there are some indications that clients from black and minority ethnic groups may experience less benefit from therapy, although not with all kinds of therapy. Nilsen et al. (2013) observed, for example, that in two studies of CBT for depression, young clients from ethnic minority backgrounds benefited less from therapy. Likewise in multisystemic therapy for conduct problems, young people who were of white ethnicity benefited more from the interventions than those from black and minority ethnic backgrounds (Van der Stouwe, Asscher, Stams, Deković, & van der Laan, 2014). One US-based study of family therapy found that young people of Hispanic ethnicity were benefiting less than African-American and European-American young people. Lin and Bratton (2015) found the opposite trend to most of these studies; children from black and minority ethnic groups benefit more from play therapy than white children.

Box 6.7   Defining gender and ethnicity

There are limitations in the research base for child and adolescent therapy when it comes to defining the effects of gender and ethnicity.

For example, when it comes to gender, this has been examined as a binary phenomenon – male/female. However gender-identity is a far more complex and fluid phenomenon than this suggests and a full range of experience has not yet been examined empirically in child and adolescent therapy.

Likewise, the categorizations of ethnicity mentioned in the studies above may seem rather crude to the reader but due to small sample sizes, studies are often only able to compare two groups of participants, for reasons of 'statistical power'. This means that participants in these (usually) US-based studies are often put into two categories – 'white ethnicity' and 'black and minority ethnicity' – and more nuanced ethnic classifications are often lost in the analysis.

A small number of studies have looked at the effects of gender and ethnicity on the formation of therapeutic alliances, and there is some evidence that this can have positive effects. One US-based study found that matching on the basis of gender led to children and young people staying in therapy for longer. This effect was particularly marked when boys were matched with male therapists. The same study looked at the effects of matching children or young people and therapists according to their ethnicity, and found that clients from black and minority ethnic groups who were matched with white therapists were more likely to drop out of therapy (Wintersteen, Janell, & Diamond, 2005). Matching young people and therapists on the basis of ethnicity has also been associated with positive therapeutic outcomes in two further studies (Halliday-Boykins, Schoenwald, & Letourneau, 2005; Yeh, Takeuchi, & Sue, 1994. as cited in Huey and Polo, 2008) – however these studies did not use **random allocation** to therapy, meaning other components that may account for the difference cannot be ruled out.

Overall, the evidence for the effects of child characteristics such as age, ethnicity and gender identity is somewhat fragmented and contradictory. Initial work seems to suggest that for the most part white children benefit more from psychotherapy than those from black and minority ethnic groups. Most of the studies from which these conclusions were drawn were carried out in the US. However, when it comes to play therapy, these effects are reversed. Lin and Bratton (2015) accounted for this as possibly related to less reliance on language in this type of therapy – which may make the therapy less culturally specific and confined. And just as play may be a more culturally flexible form of expression, it is also more accessible as a means of communication for younger children, perhaps explaining the differential effects here. Clearly more research is needed to confirm how important these demographic factors are in producing good therapy outcomes, and precisely what therapists and services may do about this.

Box 6.8   Gaps in research

There is not enough evidence yet to determine how child characteristics such as age, ethnicity and gender influence therapeutic outcomes.

Research as yet tells us little about whether children consistently benefit from gender and ethnic matching with their therapists and, if so, why this might be. For example, does this enhance the empathy of the therapist to the child's predicaments, or perhaps provide a role model to a young child? The latter would suggest that services closely match children to therapists on the basis of ethnicity and gender, whereas if the effect is better explained by enhanced therapist empathy, then there may be a role for greater education of therapists to be aware of the social factors that might be facing children of different genders and ethnicities. More research is clearly needed in this area, both qualitative and quantitative. As the authors of one review of research in this area conclude, 'the reality is that we know very little about whether gender, race, or matching . . . is related to the alliance in youth therapy' (Shirk & Karver, 2011: 84).

Acceptance of emotions and attachment styles

There is initial evidence that those young people that are judged as having more 'secure attachment' styles may benefit more from psychotherapy (Venta, Sharp, & Newlin, 2014; see Chapter 3 for a description of 'attachment'). The authors of this study assessed 194 adolescents on admission to psychiatric hospital, where they received a 'general inpatient treatment' containing components of CBT, systemic and interpersonal-psychodynamic approaches. They found that those young people coded as 'securely attached' on admission stayed in hospital less time than those rated as 'insecurely attached', and reported a greater reduction in their symptoms on discharge. They also found that the young person's capacity to accept their emotions – defined as how accepting they were of more difficult emotions, such as sadness or anger – was an important factor in change. Acceptance/non-acceptance of emotions was a **mediating variable** for the relationship between the attachment style and outcome. In other words, those who were coded as secure in their attachment patterns, but found their emotions difficult to accept did less well.

Having more than one diagnosis

There is not yet enough evidence to state conclusively whether children meeting criteria for more than one diagnosis have poorer therapy outcomes compared to children with just one diagnosis. In their review of clinical trials for psychotherapy with children and young people, Ollendick, Jarrett, Grills-Taquechel, Hovey and Wolff (2008: 1465) noted that being given more than one diagnosis was 'the rule, rather than the exception' (see also Chapter 2), but that this was not associated with poorer outcome. However, a study by Nilsen et al. (2013), reviewing therapies for anxiety and depression in children and young people, adds potential complexity to this picture. They found that those young people who were receiving therapy for depression, but were also experiencing anxiety, benefited less from their therapy. It is worth noting that the vast majority of the studies reviewed by Ollendick et al. and Nilsen et al. were of cognitive behavioural therapies, with a scattering of interpersonal therapy.

Interpersonal environment and social support

The picture is a little clearer when it comes to the young person's social environment. Several studies have found that the greater the social support surrounding the child or young person, the stronger the alliance with a therapist is likely to be (Shirk & Karver, 2011). Social support has also been linked directly with therapeutic outcomes, although there is far less research assessing this. For example, Black and Chung (2014) found that higher levels of social support led to better outcomes for young people receiving therapy for substance abuse.

Also within the realm of social relationships, those young people with more interpersonal problems are less likely to form good alliances. One particular study of young people who had been maltreated found that interpersonal problems predicted difficulties in forming a relationship with a therapist over and above the severity of their overall emotional/psychological difficulties (Eltz, Shirk, & Sarlin, 1995). Similarly, Fields, Handelsman, Karver and Bickman (2010) found that those young people judged to possess more 'social competence' formed stronger therapeutic alliances.

These findings will probably not be surprising – it follows that the more a child or young person has experienced healthy, supportive relationships and had opportunities to learn social skills, the better position they will be in to trust themselves and a therapist enough to form a bond. This, in turn, can have an influence on whether or not a child benefits from therapy as an overall experience.

What makes a good child therapist? Therapist factors

In adult psychotherapy research, it is acknowledged that although therapy helps on average around 80 per cent of people who use it, there are large differences in effectiveness *between* different therapists. This led to further enquiry into the characteristics of individual therapists, including therapist qualities such as their interpersonal skills, their direct influencing/involvement skills, and their training – and the impact of such factors on therapeutic outcomes (see Cooper, 2008 for a full discussion). This section summarizes the research that has taken place into some of these therapist characteristics in work with children and adolescents (and in some cases, their families). It is important to understand the role that these features play because as therapists, these qualities, and ways of relating, may be more in our control than some other important factors such as the characteristics of the child.

Interpersonal skills

In child therapy research, interpersonal skills have generally been defined as empathy, warmth and genuineness, which has considerable overlap with the 'core conditions' of person-centred therapy (see Chapter 7). These interpersonal skills have been linked to positive outcomes with children and adolescents. In their meta-analysis of 16 studies, Karver et al. (2006) found that counsellor interpersonal skills were quite strongly linked to therapeutic outcomes, with an effect size of 0.75 (d) (i.e. a medium effect). It is also similar to the findings in therapy with adults, where levels of therapist empathy are strongly associated with outcomes (the direction of this relationship being the more empathy from the therapist, the better the outcomes for clients – see Bohart, Elliott, Greenberg, & Watson, 2002). The difference in child and adolescent therapy is that empathy has been rarely measured separately and tends to be assessed in a package with warmth and genuineness, although one study that focused specifically on the therapist's 'accurate empathy' (as rated by parents) did identify an association with good child outcomes (Green, 1996).

Direct influencing skills/Therapist involvement

In the same review, Karver et al. (2006) found an even stronger relationship between what they termed 'therapist direct influencing skills' and outcomes. Here, the effect size was 0.87 (d, a large effect) but this was based on only five studies. This therapist quality was defined and measured as the presence of 'directive therapist behaviour', including:

- active structuring of a session;
- providing a rationale for treatment/therapy approach;
- giving guidance and instructions (Karver et al., 2006).

Box 6.9   Implications for practice

On face value, these findings may appear to contradict what was said earlier in this chapter about the importance of not being too directive with children and young people in forming good working alliances, particularly at the beginning of therapy. But if we look back to Box 6.2 the factors associated with a strong alliance are not necessarily incompatible with giving a session structure, providing guidance and instructions for any therapy tasks, and providing a rationale for therapeutic techniques and practices. Directivity, structure and instruction all are all relative terms. In addition, the studies reported in Box 6.2 are all studies of CBT, a relatively more structured approach, and these suggest that practices that are too task focused, at the expense of building a relationship, and giving a young person space to tell their story, are counterproductive. However Karver et al.'s (2006) review of therapist direct influencing skills was in the context of different types of therapies, and this suggests that there may be key moments where therapists can actively provide some instruction and explanation for therapeutic tasks, where relevant, but also actively provide signs of care and encouragement.

This interpretation is supported by other studies that have shown that children and young people seem to benefit more when a therapist shows active involvement in therapy without being controlling or domineering. In a meta-analysis of the factors involved in dropping out of therapy early, de Haan et al. (2013) found that therapists showing care and concern, and being communicative and supportive, was linked to fewer drop outs. Therapists who were described as 'directive, controlling and confronting' had significantly more clients leaving therapy early.

So should therapists be directive, or non-directive, with children? Perhaps the question itself is wrong-headed, and flexibility, rather than directivity/non-directivity per se, is a more important therapist quality. For example, one study looked at the process of therapy with children receiving CBT for anxiety disorders. They found just one therapist quality – 'therapist flexibility' – to be linked to children being much more involved in their therapy (Hudson et al., 2014). Taking the same subject from a different angle, Zack, Castonguay and Boswell (2007) found that rigid adherence to treatment protocols led to weaker alliances with children. Taken together then, we could conclude that the research suggests that therapists who work more flexibly, showing a range of interpersonal skills, are able to engage with children and young people more, potentially leading to better therapeutic outcomes.

Box 6.10   Gaps in research

Therapist 'interpersonal skills' and 'direct influencing skills' have both been associated with good therapeutic outcomes with children and young people. But how do these come together in a helping relationship – for example, how do we know when it is good to intervene, and when it is good to give a child or young person space to talk? Research that looks in detail at the therapeutic process with children and adolescents could help therapists to understand how and when to show these various qualities. But so far few such studies have been undertaken.

There are large gaps in our knowledge of whether therapist gender, age, ethnicity, training and experience, and levels of distress have an impact on the effectiveness of therapy with children and young people. For example, do adolescents prefer younger therapists because they are easier to relate to? Or older ones because they are more like a parent (or grandparent)? Are therapists who experience significant personal distress less or more able to work well with young clients? Therapist factors are a very neglected area of research in child and adolescent therapy and more enquiry is needed as a guide for therapists' training, practice, self-care and personal development.

Training

Does having therapy with a trained therapeutic professional lead to better outcomes for children and young people than when they receive help from someone without this training? As therapists, we are invested in hoping that this is the case! But interestingly enough, the findings are mixed. In a large meta-analysis of therapeutic outcomes with children and young people, 'paraprofessionals', defined as people in helping roles but with no formal mental health training, actually had better outcomes than mental health professionals (Weisz, Weiss, Han, Granger, & Morton, 1995). But in two more recent meta-analyses, trained therapeutic professionals outperformed paraprofessionals (Baskin et al., 2010; Stice, Shaw, Bohon, Marti, & Rohde, 2009). To complicate matters, some of the effects that are measured for 'paraprofessionals' involve situations where a parent, or teacher, has had a little training and/or supervision with a trained professional therapist – such as in filial play therapy (which is discussed further below in 'the role of caregivers').

Box 6.11   Gaps in research

This area is still inconclusive, and it is not yet clear whether the effects of working with para-professionals are greater if the helper is already a teacher or caregiver for the child or young person. If so, this could account for the advantage in some studies rather than the amount of training per se; but it might suggest that more therapeutic support should be provided by people who already have a relationship with a child, with mental health professionals taking a supporting role. More research is needed to compare the effects that the amount of formal training of therapists has on therapeutic outcomes with children and young people.

Session focus

There is some evidence from therapy for young people using drugs that taking a family focus in sessions, as opposed to a purely individual focus, leads to more improvement within therapy (Hogue, Dauber, Liddle, & Samuolis, 2004). The authors compared two types of therapy – individual cognitive therapy and multidimensional family therapy – finding that a family focus led to more improvements in both types of therapy. This finding is supported by a classic study that compared two therapists with better and worse outcomes (Ricks, 1974) – in that the therapist who performed better showed a greater engagement with the contexts of his clients' lives (see Box 6.12 for more on this 'Supershrink').

Box 6.12   Key studies: Supershrinks and pseudoshrinks

A fascinating study by Ricks published in 1974 aimed to shine a light on what leads some therapists to much better or worse outcomes with young people.

Ricks tracked the long-term outcomes for adolescent males who had been referred for quite severe emotional and social problems to a clinic in the US. Ricks looked at how many of these

(Continued)

(Continued)

young people had grown up to develop problems of living, including, in many cases, hospitalization for schizophrenia. What came to light through this enquiry was that the young people who had worked with two therapists in particular had very different trajectories. In Therapist A's caseload, 27 per cent had gone on to be diagnosed and hospitalized for schizophrenia, whereas 84 per cent of Therapist B's had fulfilled the same fate. Therapist A became known as 'Supershrink' and his unfortunate colleague acquired the nickname 'Pseudoshrink'.

A remarkable difference. However, how do we know that there weren't other factors that accounted for this? For example, perhaps Therapist B worked with young people with much more severe problems than Therapist A. Ricks looked at the characteristics of the two groups on entry to the service and in fact found that they were well matched in terms of their demographic characteristics and severity of difficulties. So Ricks decided to analyse the session notes of the two therapists to ascertain whether there were any differences in the way the two therapists worked with the boys. He identified the following factors that seemed to be setting Therapist A's work apart from Therapist B's:

- Therapist A gave more time to those with greater problems.
- Therapist A engaged more with the immediate problems in the social environment, while Therapist B focused on the 'intrapsychic'.
- Therapist A helped the young people develop some autonomy from their parents, while recognizing the impact on parents of this change and, at times, supporting them with the shift.
- Therapist A used 'the therapy relationship as an anchor to reality' (Ricks, 1974: 285). What Ricks meant by this was that Therapist A helped the adolescents to solve the practical problems in their lives, and also accommodated 'spontaneous' visits from them when he was needed.
- Therapist A spent more time helping the young people to think through the consequences of different courses of action.

The role of parents and caregivers

Probably one of the most important ways in which therapeutic work with children and young people is different from work with adults is the central (and often, direct) involvement of other people in the therapy. Very often, parents and caregivers are the ones who decide when and whether therapy is needed, are responsible for transporting a child or young person to therapy, and may even be the most distressed by the child's problems. Intuitively, this means that there exists a relationship between therapists and caregivers, that is moreover a very important one. The research on the whole supports this assumption, although not without some complexities.

Parent–therapist alliance

The research so far suggests that the association between the parent–therapist alliance and outcomes (i.e. amount of change in the child) varies considerably (between –0.09 to 0.67 in 10 studies) with an overall average effect size of $d = 0.11$, classed as a small effect (Karver et al., 2006). In their meta-analysis, Karver et al. (2006) note that this is a surprisingly modest effect, and suggest that there might be some methodological reasons that skew these results towards a smaller effect size. Indeed, in a later meta-analysis by McLeod (2011), which included more studies, the effect size was estimated a little higher at 0.15 – though still fairly small. The author concluded that 'the youth psychotherapy literature has a long way to go before it can match the adult literature in overall number of studies or consistency of findings. It may therefore be most appropriate to view the current findings as an important *initial estimate*' (McLeod, 2011: 614, my emphasis). This tentative language in fact characterizes many research papers in the area of 'common factors' in child and adolescent therapy.

Other (smaller) studies have suggested that the parent–therapist relationship seems to be most strongly associated with the continuation of therapy, rather than a reduction in distress (Kazdin, Holland, & Crowley, 1997; Zack et al., 2007). The implication is that if there is a weak relationship between the therapist and a caregiver, that caregiver is less likely to see the worth of their child continuing with therapy. These authors conclude that both the child–therapist and caregiver–therapist alliances are important, but for different reasons: a strong child–therapist alliance being associated with more 'symptom reduction' or therapeutic change in the child, and a strong caregiver–therapist alliance associated with lower levels of therapy drop out – thereby allowing the chance for change to happen (Kazdin et al., 1997; Zack et al., 2007).

Parental involvement in therapy

It seems that there may be on average a small but beneficial effect of involving parents/caregivers in therapy sessions, but not in all situations. One meta-analysis looked at 48 studies that compared the involvement of parents in therapy with their non-involvement. This found an average effect size of 0.27 of involving parents within therapy on the outcomes for their children (considered a small effect; Dowell & Ogles, 2010). The majority of studies in this meta-analysis were of CBT treatments, but there were 10 'non-CBT' studies included (which were mostly classed as client-centred, systemic, or psychodynamic). The effect of involving parents was in fact most apparent in these non-cognitive therapies. This suggests a beneficial effect on the child of involving their parents in therapy, particularly in more relationally oriented psychotherapies.

Evidence from the field of play therapy also supports the idea that involving caregivers may enhance the therapy for children. In some types of play therapy, parents are not only involved but actually deliver the therapy instead of a therapist. This is known as 'filial therapy' and happens alongside training and supervision by qualified therapists. One meta-analysis, containing a total of 93 studies, compared this type of therapy to others that do not involve parents in this way, finding remarkably large effect sizes for filial therapy ($d = 1.15$, as opposed to 0.72 when delivered by a mental health professional; Bratton et al., 2005). A later meta-analysis of client-centred play therapy also supports the involvement of parents and teachers (Lin & Bratton, 2015). There is, in addition, evidence that involving parents in therapy helps young people who self-injure to benefit from therapy (Glenn, Franklin, & Nock, 2015).

However, one area in which involving parents in therapy does not seem to help is in CBT for children diagnosed with anxiety (Breinholst, Esbjørn, Reinholdt-Dunne, & Stallard, 2012). In their review of 11 studies, Breinholst et al. (2012) found very mixed results and stated that the effects of involving parents were inconclusive.

Box 6.13   Gaps in research

More research is needed to find the optimum ways that parents can participate in their child's therapy, across different types of therapy, and with different types of child problems. This should include how they should be involved, and when in the process. It would be very beneficial to gather the views of parents, children and therapists about the effects of parent involvement within therapy.

There is a particular lack of evidence on parental involvement in therapies in humanistic and psychodynamic therapies and furthering knowledge in this area would be very timely.

Parental expectations

There are a handful of studies that have looked at parental attitudes to their child's therapy and the relationship this has to outcomes. A review of four studies that examined parental *willingness* to participate in treatment (as opposed to their actual level of participation; Karver et al., 2006) found a moderate relationship between parental willingness and therapeutic change in the child, at an effect size of $d = 0.65$. A related concept, parent expectations of therapy, was examined by Nock and Kazdin (2001). In this study, the children of those parents with very high expectations of what therapy could achieve, *and very low expectations*, were less likely to drop out of therapy early, and attended the greatest number of sessions overall. It was those parents with expectations somewhere in the middle that were most at risk of dropping out of therapy early, and attending fewer sessions. The authors described this as a **curvilinear relationship** between expectations and outcomes (see Figure 6.1).

Perceived barriers

The same study by Nock and Kazdin (2001) also looked at the barriers faced by parents to their child participating in therapy. Barriers are things like obstacles in

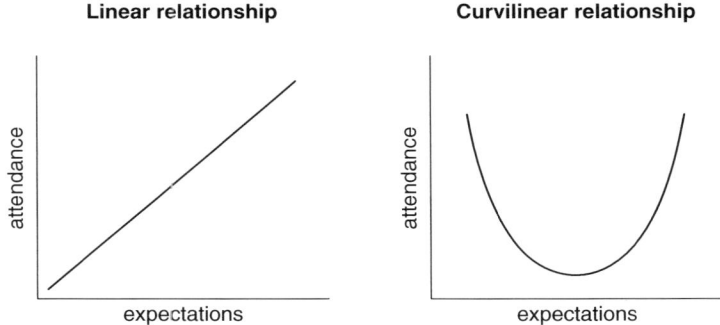

Figure 6.1 Linear and curvilinear relationships between parent expectations of therapy and attendance

getting to therapy (such as demands of employment or transport problems), or a weak alliance with a therapist. They found a **linear relationship** between parental expectations of therapy and subsequent barriers – parents with low expectations of therapy experienced more barriers to their child participating. These barriers decreased as their expectations for the therapy improved.

In turn, parent-perceived barriers have been shown to significantly predict therapeutic outcomes in children and young people referred for 'antisocial behaviour' (Kazdin & Wassell, 2000) as well as dropping out of therapy (Kazdin et al., 1997). Kazdin and Wassell (2000) showed that those parents who perceived the therapy as making demands on them, and saw the therapy as not being particularly relevant to their child's problems, had children who experienced less therapeutic change. In this study, perceived barriers had an effect size on therapeutic change in the medium range ($r = 0.32$, a Cohen's d of around 50; Kazdin & Wassell, 2000).

Becker, Lee, Daleiden, Lindsey, Brandt and Chorpita (2015) examined the features of therapies that managed to successfully engage families and found that those therapies and services that 'promoted accessibility' (such as by providing transport or childcare), and that took time to assess barriers to attendance, achieved much greater engagement overall in terms of attendance and levels of participation.

Parenting styles

There has been a small amount of research looking at parenting practices –how a caregiver is looking after a young person, and relating to them – and whether these practices may be enhancing or detracting from therapeutic effects. A review of four studies found that 'positive parenting behaviours' were a mediator of change in young people in therapy for substance use (Black & Chung, 2014). But what does 'improved parenting' look like? From the review, it is not clear but Henderson, Rowe, Dakof, Hawes and Liddle (2009) evaluated the level of 'parental monitoring' of their children over time, while Winters, Lee, Botzet, Fahnhorst and Nicholson (2014) cited more 'consistent discipline', 'parental monitoring' and 'positive parenting' as improving therapeutic outcomes with such children.

In the absence of research with other types of child and adolescent problems, we cannot conclude that such parenting styles would be beneficial for everyone. For example, increased parental monitoring of a child/adolescent, while perhaps leading to less opportunity for substance abuse, could be experienced as intrusive and anxiety provoking and make other problems worse.

Kazdin et al. (1997) looked at what parents reported about their parenting practices before therapy, and the links to dropping out. They found that parents who reported the use of harsh child-rearing practices prior to therapy were much more likely to drop out of therapy. This research concerned therapy for children aged 3–14 diagnosed with antisocial behaviour. In a similar vein, Gorin (1993) measured the frequency of 'psychological punishment' of children in therapy by their parents. This was defined as parent actions such as guilt induction or withdrawal of privileges to punish the child. This, the author found, unsurprisingly, was associated with worse therapeutic outcomes for children.

Box 6.14   Gaps in research

There is a real need for more detail about what types of parenting practices may be developed during therapy to produce better outcomes for children. Qualitative research would have a crucial role here in examining the specifics of what these 'improved' parent–child interactions might involve. This would enable more specific knowledge to be gathered about exactly how parents can facilitate the impact of therapy for their children, and in turn highlight the kinds of parenting practices that therapists might want to encourage.

Parental perceptions of severity of their child's difficulties

A small cluster of studies of therapy with children with antisocial behavioural problems found that parental perception of the severity of these problems was correlated with different types of outcomes. For example, those that saw their children as having more severe problems were more likely to drop out of therapy (Kazdin et al., 1997), have low expectations for therapy (Nock & Kazdin, 2001), and their children were likely to experience less therapeutic change overall (Kazdin & Wassell, 2000). In addition, the parents of older children had lower expectations for the utility of therapy (Nock & Kazdin, 2001).

Parental characteristics affecting the outcomes of child therapy

A few studies, all focused on children diagnosed with oppositional and antisocial behaviour, have looked at how characteristics of parents, that could also be considered to be pre-treatment characteristics, affect outcomes for children and young people. What follows is a list of demographic factors of parents and the therapy factors they have been correlated with:

- Socio-economic disadvantage – linked to low expectations, dropping out, and less therapeutic change
- Ethnic minority group status – low expectations, dropping out
- Single parent households – dropping out
- Younger parents – dropping out.

(Compiled from Kazdin & Wassell, 2000; Kazdin et al., 1997; Nock & Kazdin., 2001.)

In addition, parental stress and depression have been linked to low expectations for therapy and less therapeutic change in their children (Kazdin, 1999; Kazdin & Wassell, 2000; Nock & Kazdin, 2001), as has parent-reported quality of life (Kazdin & Wassell, 2000).

One qualitative study attempted to get at some of the reasons why treatment is ended early by parents, by interviewing the parents of children who completed a course of therapy, as well as the parents of those who left therapy early (Attride-Stirling, 2004). They found that what characterized the accounts of non-completing parents was a picture of families who were simply overwhelmed by multiple difficulties, where getting their child to therapy appointments became an additional burden. For example, some parents' employers were not flexible about the hours they worked and this made it impossible for some families to take their child to appointments without experiencing employment difficulties or less income, which would in turn create more problems for the entire family. Despite these findings, three studies have found that even if a family had several of these pre-treatment 'risk factors' for dropping out, a good experience of therapy with few barriers cancelled the effects of these multiple disadvantages (Kazdin, 1999; Kazdin & Wassell, 2000; Kazdin et al., 1997).

The role of therapist–family alliance

Some studies of therapy involving other members of the family have measured the therapeutic alliance between the family and a therapist, finding a medium effect size. In a meta-analysis of five studies, the correlation between the family's alliance with a therapist and outcomes for the child reached an effect size of $d = 0.45$ (Karver et al., 2006). It will be remembered that this is higher than the alliance with parents (which was $d = 0.22$), although it is based on fewer studies, which could mean that this is less accurate. The authors also found that this alliance was correlated strongly with treatment satisfaction ($d = 1.42$) in one study, and in another, had a small effect on treatment completion (0.35; see Karver et al., 2006).

Box 6.15   Implications for practice

The research evidence on parent/caregiver and family factors all points towards the importance of therapists engaging beyond the individual child to the context of their life.

In particular, the social and economic context of therapy is very important. When looking at some of the barriers faced by parents and families in enabling their child to attend therapy, there is a role for employers, and wider society, in reducing some of these barriers, to avoid the 'poor becoming poorer'. At a service level, something as simple as providing transport to sessions can significantly promote the accessing of therapy by those who need it most. This has obvious implications for the need for enough state funding for therapy services.

The evidence suggests that some work can also be done at the psychological and relational level to reduce the impact of these barriers. The research points towards the importance of spending time with parents/caregivers to understand their expectations of therapy, to explain to them clearly what therapy can and cannot offer, and the rationale for the therapy approach in terms of their child's problems. It seems particularly important to have these conversations with those parents who appear to be ambivalent about the value of therapy – with neither high nor low expectations for what it could achieve.

The setting of therapy

We have seen so far that the family and social setting in which children and young people live is important in impeding or enhancing the impact that psychotherapy can have. Does the service setting in which therapy takes place, such as the school, or a clinic, influence how beneficial therapy is for children and young people?

Where should therapy be offered?

For a long time, it has been observed that the effectiveness of child and adolescent therapy achieved in clinical trials (where, as Chapter 4 explains, the conditions are often more tightly controlled than in 'real world' settings) seemed to decline once rolled out into other settings, such as schools (Verdeli, Mufson, Lee, & Keith, 2006). However recent evidence has begun to challenge this assumption, finding equivalent effects of delivering therapy in schools. Two recent meta-analyses of school-based therapies have found effect sizes of 0.44 and 0.45 (Baskin et al., 2010; Reese, 2010). This is in-between the estimated effects for all types of child and adolescent therapy (0.54; Weisz et al., 1995) and those specifically for depression (0.34; Weisz et al., 1995). Interpersonal psychotherapy for adolescents diagnosed with depression has also been found to be equally effective when delivered in schools (Mufson, 2010). This was determined by comparing the effect sizes from school-based therapies delivered by community clinicians with those from trials. However, another meta-analysis has found that cognitive behavioural therapies for young people with antisocial behavioural problems were more effective in clinical settings than in schools (McCart, Priester, Davies, & Azen, 2006), and a recent study of CBT indicates that young people receiving this in university-research settings formed better alliances with their therapists than those attending a community mental health clinic (McLeod, Jensen-Doss, Tully, Southam-Gerow, Weisz, & Kendall, 2016).

When it comes to play therapy, which has compared effects across a number of settings, children seemed to benefit the most from this therapy when it was delivered in crisis settings and residential settings, as opposed to schools or outpatient clinics (Bratton et al., 2005). Crisis and residential settings included hospitals, prisons, domestic violence shelters and services following natural disasters. If this finding holds for other types of therapy and children, it may have implications for services with waiting lists.

In sum, there are indications that offering therapy in community settings may not mean that we have to compromise on success rates. However, there is little research that directly compares the same therapy when delivered in multiple settings, with a randomized sample of participants – an RCT, but instead of comparing therapies, comparing the same therapy offered in different settings. The study by McLeod et al. (2016) is an exception here, and suggests that in CBT at least, young people may form better alliances in university-research settings. More research of this kind would give us a better picture of what type of setting leads to the best outcomes. But there are also other things to consider – such as the acceptability of the different settings to children, young people and their families. There may be obvious advantages of offering therapy in the community which are not captured by simple measures of clinical change, such as how much stigma is attached (Donald, Rickwood, & Carey, 2014), as well as how easy it may be for children, young people and their families to access these services. These two factors address some of the barriers to participation that influence caregiver engagement in their child's therapy.

Online and telephone therapy

There is preliminary evidence that delivering therapy to adolescents online and over the telephone may be just as effective as face-to-face work. Slone, Reese and McClellan

(2012) reviewed studies that used video-conferencing technology, online chat forums and the telephone to deliver therapy. They found no significant differences with face-to-face work and, moreover, with some types of problems, these alternative modes of delivery may even yield better results. For example, Fridrici and Lohaus (2009, as cited in Slone et al., 2012) looked at the delivery of an online CBT programme for anxiety and stress. They compared the outcomes of those in three groups: children who accessed the programme online at school, those who accessed it online at home, and those receiving face-to-face therapy. Those with the biggest gains were the children who used the programme online at school, although interestingly those receiving face-to-face therapy reported the highest levels of satisfaction with the service.

A common concern about the use of alternative modes of delivery to face-to-face therapies, in particular internet-based therapies, is that this will interfere with the formation of a strong therapeutic alliance – or even bypass the formation of a therapeutic relationship altogether, as is the case in some online self-help interventions. There are very few studies that delve into this area, but one study comparing therapy delivered face-to-face with both video-conferencing and speakerphone produced some interesting findings. The therapy was a type of family therapy for families with children suffering from epilepsy. Glueckauf, Fritz, Eklund-Johnson, Liss, Dages and Carney (2002) found that not only were outcomes similar across the three modes of delivery, but so too was the quality of the therapeutic alliance as rated by the families themselves (as cited in Slone et al., 2012). It seems that it might not be necessary to be in the same room as a client to form a good therapeutic relationship with them. A study looking at therapy via text message also found that children reported 'a relational connection' with the therapist, despite the fact that they did not know who was replying to their texts (Gibson & Cartwright, 2014). They also reported valuing the privacy, control and autonomy that the service offered.

Box 6.16   Gaps in research

There is not yet definitive evidence to suggest which setting leads to the best outcomes for children and young people. More studies are needed to directly compare the effects of different settings on the delivery and effectiveness of therapy. Qualitative research is also needed to gauge the impact and acceptability of therapy in a range of settings to children, young people and families. The evidence for online therapy is in its infancy, but initial studies indicate that alternative modes of delivery may be just as beneficial for some children. The advantage of this type of therapy is that it may overcome some of the barriers to accessing services discussed above, so further research is clearly needed.

Conclusion

The research into common factors in youth therapy is still in its infancy, with some areas embryonic or maybe even just a twinkle in the eye of a therapy researcher. Putting together the sometimes patchy findings reported here with nothing else would lead to a very odd kind of practice. This chapter is written in the spirit that these findings can inform our practice rather than dictate it. For example, they can aid our reflection on how our work is developing with each child or young person in our care. When designing new services, they may inform our decisions on what elements might be important to include to maximize service use by children and families.

Taking the findings for common factors in youth psychotherapy all together, perhaps there are some things we can be fairly sure of. They suggest that it is crucial to see beyond the individual child or young person in successful therapeutic work. This involves therapists being aware of the impact of the child or young person's everyday lived environment – the barriers that they and their caregivers may be facing to even access therapy. But it also involves being tuned into relationships. The therapy relationship, which needs to be mutually established, and formed by a degree of willingness and respect from both therapist and child, is just as important as it is in adult therapies (although, as a medium effect size, this is clearly not the whole picture). The same process also needs to occur with the parents/caregivers in those situations where the child's attendance is dependent on these adults seeing the worth of their child's therapy, and of the therapist. The research is also beginning to show the ways in which therapists can engage young people, and their caregivers, more in the process. This gives therapists the possibility to work on their own skills in order to maximize engagement and outcomes with children and young people – in particular, their interpersonal skills such as warmth, genuineness and empathy, and their ability to offer structure and guidance on therapy tasks.

Summary of key findings

- The quality of the therapy relationship is moderately related to outcomes in child and adolescent therapy – in both relationally focused and non-relationally focused therapies.
- The strength of the therapeutic alliance is also associated with how much benefit is obtained from therapy – and this is particularly the case when working with younger children.
- A strong working alliance with caregivers is associated with continuation of therapy – thereby giving children and young people more opportunity to receive the beneficial effects of therapy.
- Children and young people who are more involved in their therapy, engaged, show autonomy and see reasons for changing, are more likely to benefit from therapy.
- Many children and young people do not know what to expect from therapy.
- The amount of social support a child or young person has is related to how much they change in therapy.
- The ways a therapist relates to children and young people are linked to outcomes – in particular their capacity to offer empathy, warmth, genuineness, flexibility, involvement, guidance and instruction.
- Therapists who engage with the interpersonal world of the child/young person, particularly with their parents and caregivers, rather than taking a solely individual focus, are more likely to achieve success.
- The expectations that parents/caregivers have about therapy and the barriers they perceive about participating have an impact on outcomes for their children.
- The amount of adversity that families as a whole are facing affects the benefits that children and young people obtain from therapy.
- There may be a small but beneficial effect of involving parents/caregivers in their child's therapy sessions – but not for all types of therapy or for all children/young people and families.

Recommended reading

Karver, M. S., Handelsman, J. B., Fields, S., & Bickman, L. (2006). Meta-analysis of therapeutic relationship variables in youth and family therapy: The evidence for different relationship variables in the child and adolescent treatment outcome literature. *Clinical Psychology Review*, 26, 50–65. This journal article is the broadest review available of the research evidence for different common factors in child and adolescent therapies, including 'therapist influencing skills' and 'parent–therapist alliance'.

Questions for reflection

- Were any of the findings reported here surprising to you?
- If so, why was this the case? Do you think they will change anything about how you work?
- What other therapist factors do you think could be important in working with children and young people? What things about yourself do you think enhance, or obstruct your work, and why do you think this is the case?

References

Adelman, H. S., Kaser-Boyd, N., & Taylor, L. (1984). Children's participation in consent for psychotherapy and their subsequent response to treatment. *Journal of Clinical Child Psychology*, 13, 170–178.

Asay, T. P., & Lambert, M. J. (1999). The empirical case for the common factors in therapy. In M. A. Hubble, B. L. Duncan, & S. D. Miller (Eds.), *The heart and soul of change: What works in therapy* (pp. 23–55). Washington, DC: American Psychological Association.

Attride-Stirling, J. (2004). Factors influencing parental engagement in a community child and adolescent mental health service: A qualitative comparison of completers and non-completers. *Clinical Child Psychology and Psychiatry*, 9, 347–361.

Baskin, T. W., Slaten, C. D., Crosby, N. R., Pufahl, T., Schneller, C. L., & Ladell, M. (2010). Efficacy of counseling and psychotherapy in schools: A meta-analytic review of treatment outcome studies. *The Counseling Psychologist*, 38, 878–903.

Becker, K. D., Lee, B. R., Daleiden, E. L., Lindsey, M., Brandt, N. E., & Chorpita, B. F. (2015). The common elements of engagement in children's mental health services: Which elements for which outcomes? *Journal of Clinical Child and Adolescent Psychology*, 53, 37–41.

Berg, D. R. (1999). An examination of the relationship between process variables and outcome indicators in the therapeutic use of play with children. Unpublished doctoral dissertation, University of Illinois.

Black, J. J., & Chung, T. (2014). Mechanisms of change in adolescent substance use treatment: How does treatment work? *Substance Abuse*, 35, 344–351.

Bohart, A. C., Elliott, R., Greenberg, L. S., & Watson, J. C. (2002). Empathy. In J. C. Norcross (Ed.), *Psychotherapy relationships that work: Therapist contributions and responsiveness to patients* (pp. 89–108). New York: Oxford University Press.

Bordin, E. (1979). The generalizability of the psychoanalytic concept of the working alliance. *Psychotherapy: Theory, Research and Practice*, 16, 252–260.

Bratton, S. C., Ray, D., Rhine, T., & Jones, L. (2005). The efficacy of play therapy with children: A meta-analytic review of treatment outcomes. *Professional Psychology: Research and Practice*, 36, 376–390.

Breinholst, S., Esbjørn, B. H., Reinholdt-Dunne, M. L., & Stallard, P. (2012). CBT for the treatment of child anxiety disorders: A review of why parental involvement has not enhanced outcomes. *Journal of Anxiety Disorders*, 26, 416–424.

Carlberg, G., Thorén, A., Billström, S., & Odhammar, F. (2009). Children's expectations and experiences of psychodynamic child psychotherapy. *Journal of Child Psychotherapy*, 35, 175–193.

Chu, B. C., & Kendall, P. C. (2009). Therapist responsiveness to child engagement: Flexibility within manual-based CBT for anxious youth. *Journal of Clinical Psychology*, 65, 736–754.

Cooper, M (2008). *Essential research findings in counselling and psychotherapy: The facts are friendly.* London: Sage.

Creed, T. A., & Kendall, P. C. (2005). Therapist alliance-building behavior within a cognitive-behavioral treatment for anxiety in youth. *Journal of Consulting and Clinical Psychology*, 73, 498 - 511

de Haan, A. M., Boon, A. E., de Jong, J. T. V. M., Hoeve, M., Vermeiren, R. R. J. M., Jones, P., & Zetterqvist Nelson, K. (2013). Client-identified important events in psychotherapy: Interactional structures and practices. *Psychotherapy Research* , 33, 698–711.

Donald, I. N., Rickwood, D. J., & Carey, T. A. (2014). Understanding therapeutic change in young people: A pressing research agenda. *Journal of Psychotherapy Integration*, 24, 313–322.

Dowell, K., & Ogles, B. M. (2010). The effects of parent participation on child psychotherapy outcome: A meta-analytic review. *Journal of Clinical Child and Adolescent Psychology*, 39, 151–162.

Eltz, M. J., Shirk, S. R., & Sarlin, N. (1995). Alliance formation and treatment outcome among maltreated adolescents. *Child Abuse & Neglect*, 19, 419–431.

Estrada, A., & Russell, R. (1999). The development of Child Psychotherapy Process Scales (CPPS). *Psychotherapy Research*, 9, 154–166.

Fields, S., Handelsman, J., Karver, M. S., & Bickman, L. (2010). Youth and parent predictors of therapeutic alliance.

Fitzpatrick, M., & Irannejad, S. (2008). Adolescent readiness for change and the working alliance in counseling. *Journal of Counseling and Development*, 86, 438–445.

Freud, A. (1946). *The psycho-analytical treatment of children.* London: Imago.

Fridrici, M., & Lohaus, A. (2009). Stress-prevention in secondary schools: Online-versus face-to-face-training. *Health Education*, 109, 299–313.

Gibson, K., & Cartwright, C. (2014). Young people's experiences of mobile phone text counselling: Balancing connection and control. *Children and Youth Services Review*, 43, 96–104.

Glenn, C. R., Franklin, J. C., & Nock, M. K. (2015). Evidence-based psychosocial treatments for self-injurious thoughts and behaviors in youth. *Journal of Clinical Child and Adolescent Psychology*, 44, 1–29.

Glueckauf, R. L., Fritz, S. P., Ecklund-Johnson, E. P., Liss, H. J., Dages, P., & Carney, P. (2002). Videoconferencing-based family counseling for rural teenagers with epilepsy: Phase 1 findings. *Rehabilitation Psychology*, 47, 49–72.

Gorin, S. S. (1993). The prediction of child psychotherapy outcome: Factors specific to treatment. *Psychotherapy: Theory, Research, Practice, Training*, 30, 152–158.

Gorin, S. S., & Gorin, S. S. (1993). The prediction of child psychotherapy outcome: Factors specific to treatment. *Psychotherapy*, 30, 152–158.

Green, J. M. (1996). Engagement and empathy: A pilot study of the therapeutic alliance in outpatient child psychiatry. *Child and Adolescent Mental Health*, 1, 130–138.

Halliday-Boykins, C. A., Schoenwald, S. K., & Letourneau, E. J. (2005). Caregiver–therapist ethnic similarity predicts youth outcomes from an empirically based treatment. *Journal of Consulting and Clinical Psychology*, 73, 808–818.

Henderson, C. E., Rowe, C. L., Dakof, G., Hawes, S. W., & Liddle, H. (2009). Parenting practices as mediators of treatment effects in an early-intervention trial of multidimensional family therapy. *The American Journal of Drug and Alcohol Abuse*, 35, 220–226.

Hogue, A., Dauber, S., Liddle, H., & Samuolis, J. (2004). Linking session focus to treatment outcome in evidence-based treatments for adolescent substance abuse. *Psychotherapy*, 41, 83–96.

Horvath, A., & Greenberg, L. (1989). Development and validation of the Working Alliance Inventory. *Journal of Counseling Psychology*, 36, 223–233.

Hudson, J. L., Kendall, P. C., Chu, B. C., Gosch, E., Martin, E., Taylor, A., & Knight, A. (2014). Child involvement, alliance, and therapist flexibility: Process variables in cognitive-behavioural therapy for anxiety disorders in childhood. *Behaviour Research and Therapy*, 52, 1–8.

Huey Jr, S. J., & Polo, A. J. (2008). Evidence-based psychosocial treatments for ethnic minority youth. *Journal of Clinical Child & Adolescent Psychology*, 37, 262–301.

Jungbluth, N. J., & Shirk, S. R. (2009). Therapist strategies for building involvement in cognitive-behavioral therapy for adolescent depression. *Journal of Consulting and Clinical Psychology*, 77, 1179–1184.

Karver, M. S., Handelsman, J. B., Fields, S., & Bickman, L. (2005). A theoretical model of common process factors in youth and family therapy. *Mental Health Services Research*, 7, 35–51.

Karver, M. S., Handelsman, J. B., Fields, S., & Bickman, L. (2006). Meta-analysis of therapeutic relationship variables in youth and family therapy: The evidence for different relationship variables in the child and adolescent treatment outcome literature. *Clinical Psychology Review*, 26, 50–65.

Kazdin, A. (1999). Barriers to treatment participation and therapeutic change among children referred for conduct disorder. *Journal of Clinical Child Psychology*, 28, 137–150.

Kazdin, E., & Wassell, G. (2000). Predictors of barriers to treatment and therapeutic change in outpatient therapy for antisocial children and their families. *Mental Health Services Research*, 2, 27–40.

Kazdin, E., Holland, L., & Crowley, M. (1997). Family experience of barriers to treatment and premature termination from child therapy. *Journal of Consulting and Clinical Psychology*, 65, 453–463.

Kendall, P. C., Hudson, J. L., Gosch, E., Flannery-Schroeder, E., & Suveg, C. (2009). Cognitive-behavioral therapy for anxiety-disordered youth: Secondary outcomes from a randomized clinical trial evaluating child and family modalities. *Journal of Anxiety Disorders*, 23, 341–349.

Killips, C., Cooper, M., Freire, E. S., & McGinnis, S. (2012). Motivation as a predictor of outcomes in school-based humanistic counselling. *Counselling and Psychotherapy Research*, 12, 93–99.

Labouliere, C. D., Reyes, J. P., Shirk, S., & Karver, M. (2015). Therapeutic alliance with depressed adolescents: predictor or outcome? Disentangling temporal confounds to understand early improvement. *Journal of Clinical Child and Adolescent Psychology*. Available online: doi: 10.1080/15374416.2015.1041594

Lin, Y., & Bratton, S. C. (2015). A meta-analytic review of child centered play therapy approaches. *Journal of Counseling and Development*, 93, 45–58.

McCart, M. R., Priester, P. E., Davies, W. H., & Azen, R. (2006). Differential effectiveness of behavioral parent-training and cognitive-behavioral therapy for antisocial youth: A meta-analysis. *Journal of Abnormal Child Psychology*, 34, 527–543.

McLaughlin, C., Holliday, C., Clarke, B., & Ilie, S. (2013). Research on counselling and psychotherapy with children and young people: A systematic scoping review of the evidence for its effectiveness from 2003–2011. Project Report. British Association for Counselling and Psychotherapy, Lutterworth.

McLeod, B. D. (2011). The relation of the alliance with outcomes in youth psychotherapy: A meta-analysis. *Clinical Psychology Review*, 31, 603–616.

McLeod, B. D., Jensen-Doss, A., Tully, C. B., Southam-Gerow, M. A., Weisz, J. R., & Kendall, P. C. (2016). The role of setting versus treatment type in alliance within youth therapy. *Journal of Consulting and Clinical Psychology*, 84, 453-464.

Midgley, N., Holmes, J., Parkinson, S., Stapley, E., Eatough, V., & Target, M. (2016). 'Just like talking to someone about like shit in your life and stuff, and they help you': Hopes and expectations for therapy among depressed adolescents. *Psychotherapy Research*, 26, 11–21.

Miller, S., Wampold, B., & Varhely, K. (2008). Direct comparisons of treatment modalities for youth disorders: A meta-analysis. *Psychotherapy Research*, 18, 5–14.

Mufson, L. (2010). Interpersonal psychotherapy for depressed adolescents (IPT-A): Extending the reach from academic to community settings. *Child and Adolescent Mental Health*, 15, 66–72.

Nilsen, T. S., Eisemann, M., & Kvernmo, S. (2013). Predictors and moderators of outcome in child and adolescent anxiety and depression: A systematic review of psychological treatment studies. *European Child and Adolescent Psychiatry*, 22, 69–87.

Nock, M. K., & Kazdin, A. E. (2001). Parent expectancies for child therapy: Assessment and relation to participation in treatment. *Journal of Child and Family Studies*, 10, 155–180.

Ollendick, T. H., Jarrett, M. A., Grills-Taquechel, A. E., Hovey, L. D., & Wolff, J. C. (2008). Comorbidity as a predictor and moderator of treatment outcome in youth with anxiety, affective, attention deficit/hyperactivity disorder, and oppositional/conduct disorders. *Clinical Psychology Review*, 28, 1447–1471.

Proctor, G. (2014). *Ethics and values in counselling and psychotherapy*. London: Sage.

Reese, R. J. (2010). Effectiveness of school-based psychotherapy: A meta-analysis of dissertation research. *Journal of Adolescence*, 74, 274–283.

Ricks, D. F. (1974). Supershrink: Methods of a therapist judged successful on the basis of adult outcomes of adolescent patients. In D. F. Ricks, M. F. Roff, A. Thomas, D. F. Ricks, M. F. Roff, & A. Thomas (Eds.), *Life history research in psychopathology* (Vol. 3, pp. 275–297). Minneapolis: University of Minnesota Press.

Rogers, C. R. (1957). The necessary and sufficient conditions of therapeutic personality change. *Journal of Consulting Psychology*, 21, 95–103. Reprinted in H. Kirscenbaum & V. Henderson (Eds.) (1990), *The Carl Rogers Reader* (pp. 219–235). London: Constable.

Sagen, S. H., Hummelsund, D., & Binder, P. E. (2013). Feeling accepted: A phenomenological exploration of adolescent patients' experiences of the relational qualities that enable them to express themselves freely. *European Journal of Psychotherapy and Counselling*, 15, 53–75.

Shirk, S. R., & Karver, M. (2003). Prediction of treatment outcome from relationship variables in child and adolescent therapy: A meta-analytic review. *Journal of Consulting and Clinical Psychology*, 71, 452–464.

Shirk, S., & Karver, M. S. (2011). Alliance in child and adolescent psychotherapy. In J. Norcross (Ed.), *Psychotherapy relationships that work*. Oxford: Oxford University Press.

Shirk, S. R., & Saiz, C. (1992). The therapeutic alliance in child therapy: Clinical, empirical, and developmental perspectives. *Development and Psychopathology*, 4, 713–728.

Shirk, S. R., Karver, M. S., & Brown, R. (2011). The alliance in child and adolescent psychotherapy. *Psychotherapy*, 48, 17–24.

Slone, N. C., Reese, R. J., & McClellan, M. J. (2012). Telepsychology outcome research with children and adolescents: A review of the literature. *Psychological Services*, 9, 272–292.

Stice, E., Shaw, H., Bohon, C., Marti, C. N., & Rohde, P. (2009). A meta-analytic review of depression prevention programs for children and adolescents: Factors that predict magnitude of intervention effects. *Journal of Consulting and Clinical Psychology*, 77, 486–503.

Target, M., & Fonagy, P. (1994). The efficacy of child psychoanalysis for children: Prediction of outcome in a developmental context. *Journal of the American Academy of Child and Adolescent Psychiatry*, 33, 1134–1144.

Van der Stouwe, T., Asscher, J. J., Stams, G. J. J., Deković, M., & van der Laan, P. H. (2014). The effectiveness of Multisystemic Therapy (MST): A meta-analysis. *Clinical Psychology Review*, 34, 468–481.

Venta, A., Sharp, C., & Newlin, E. (2014). A descriptive study of symptom change as a function of attachment and emotion regulation in a naturalistic adolescent inpatient setting. *European Child and Adolescent Psychiatry*, 24, 95–104.

Verdeli, H., Mufson, L., Lee, L., & Keith, J. A. (2006). Review of evidence-based psychotherapies for pediatric mood and anxiety disorders. *Current Psychiatry Reviews*, 2, 395–421.

Watsford, C., & Rickwood, D. (2014). Young people's expectations, preferences, and experiences of therapy: Effects on clinical outcome, service use, and help-seeking intentions. *Clinical Psychologist*, 18, 43–51.

Watsford, C., Rickwood, D., & Vanags, T. (2013). Exploring young people's expectations of a youth mental health care service. *Early Intervention in Psychiatry*, 7, 131–137.

Weisz, J., Weiss, B., Han, S., Granger, D., & Morton, T. (1995). Effects of psychotherapy with children and adolescents revisited: A meta-analysis of treatment outcome studies. *Psychological Bulletin*, 117, 450–468.

Weitkamp, K., Klein, E., & Midgley, N. (2016). The experience of depression: A qualitative study of adolescents with depression entering psychotherapy. *Global Qualitative Nursing Research*, 3, 1–12.

Winters, K. C., Lee, S., Botzet, A., Fahnhorst, T., & Nicholson, A. (2014). One-year outcomes and mediators of a brief intervention for drug abusing adolescents. *Psychology of Addictive Behaviors*, 28, 464–474.

Wintersteen, M., Janell, L. M., & Diamond, G. S. (2005). Do gender and racial differences between patient and therapist affect therapeutic alliance and treatment retention in adolescents? *Professional Psychology: Research and Practice*, 36(4), 400–412.

Yeh, M., Takeuchi, D. T., & Sue, S. (1994). Asian-American children treated in the mental health system: A comparison of parallel and mainstream outpatient service centers. *Journal of Clinical Child Psychology*, 23, 5–12.

Zack, S. E., Castonguay, L. G., & Boswell, J. F. (2007). Youth working alliance: A core clinical construct in need of empirical maturity. *Harvard Review of Psychiatry*, 15, 278–288.

7

WHAT LEADS TO CHANGE? II. THERAPEUTIC TECHNIQUES AND PRACTICES WITH CHILDREN AND YOUNG PEOPLE

JACQUELINE HAYES AND CLARE BRUNST

This chapter discusses

- Empirical **research** into d fferent techniques and practices used in child and adolescent therapy
- Techniques and practices associated with therapies that are:

  - Cognitive and behavioural
  - Humanistic
  - Psychodynamic
  - Arts and play
  - Narrative

- Generic therapeutic techniques, not aligned to particular schools of therapy

Introduction

This chapter is about research that explores how therapy takes place with children and young people, with a specific focus on the techniques and practices that therapists use, and the contributions these make to therapeutic change. Techniques are systematic ways of structuring therapy, introducing particular activities or conversational moves, that are underpinned by theory and training. Examples that are explored below include using mindfulness in therapy, or cognitive restructuring. But we also use the term 'practices' in order to encompass those systematic ways of responding to children and young people that might reflect the psychological climate a therapist is aiming to create – such as the attitudinal conditions in client-centred therapy, or awareness of countertransference in psychodynamic therapy – or the media a therapist may use (for example, art, music or play).

Techniques and practices are in some way dependent on the training of the therapist and the particular theories they are using to guide their practice. Since therapies tend to have different models of research and the studies reported on in this chapter use a wide range of methodologies, we are not encouraging direct comparisons between them. Rather, we would like to highlight what the different schools of therapy are doing to investigate their techniques and practices, to give the reader a flavour of what is being investigated in this area, and what some of the preliminary results are. Since, in some estimates, techniques and practices in child and adolescent therapy may be contributing as much to change as the therapeutic alliance (Miller, Wampold, & Varhely, 2008; see Chapter 6 for a discussion of the alliance), we think this survey has direct relevance to those working with children.

In this chapter we cover research on the relative power, or **efficacy** of different techniques and practices, where this research exists (the research is far behind that of adult therapies, at least in terms of volume). Efficacy is usually determined, as Chapter 6 reports, by a **quantitative** measure of functioning/symptomatology that is applied before and after the technique. However, different techniques and practices may have different aims than symptom reduction: for example, greater insight or existential meaning – which somewhat problematizes the idea of one-size-fits-all efficacy measures. Equally important to the study of therapeutic change is reaching an understanding of how and when techniques are used, their acceptability to the children and young people involved, and what their consequences are, in the fullest sense of that word. This means going beyond whether a technique results in a reduction of distress or symptomatology on outcome measures to consider the experience of the technique and perhaps the more qualitative changes that can occur as a result. In this way, research may show us exactly how therapy in the 'real world' deviates from its theoretical or manualized versions, why this could be the case, and may even allow us to reach a better understanding of the ethical dimensions of practice.

It is not always clear exactly where a technique belongs, and not all readers may agree with the way the techniques and practices are categorized below. For example, who is to say which school of therapy 'owns' relaxation – this technique is used widely in different schools of therapy but we could just as easily associate it with 'folk' psychology and ancient traditions from different parts of the world. Nevertheless, the headings used below aim to reflect broadly the theory or paradigm that the technique tends to be studied within – e.g. psychoeducation as a technique tends to be studied in trials of CBT. The chapter begins with an overview of cognitive behavioural techniques, moving to humanistic, psychodynamic, arts and play, and narrative, before ending with techniques and practices that tend to be found across multiple approaches.

Cognitive and behavioural

Graded exposure

A large volume of research has examined the use of exposure techniques with children and young people experiencing anxiety. The technique usually involves creating a safe environment in which a person can progressively overcome the anxiety and avoidance behaviours that maintain fears or phobias. According to a recent review, which looked at 32 instances where researchers compared exposure techniques to other techniques in therapy for children with obsessive-compulsive disorder or specific phobias, exposure led to decreased anxiety with a large **effect size**. The authors concluded that exposure is a 'well established treatment' for anxiety in children and young people and is among those techniques with the 'best support' (Higa-McMillan, Francis, Rith-Najarian, & Chorpita, 2015). The use of graded exposure has also been shown to be helpful in therapy with children and young people experiencing post-traumatic stress (see Cohen, Berliner, & Mannarino, 2000; Smith, Yule, Persia, Tranah, Dalgleish, & Clark, 2007), and of particular help with younger children (Peris et al., 2015). However research has not yet established whether exposure is effective for other problems – for example, its use does not seem to have a relationship to outcomes when used with children and young people with anger issues (Sukhodolsky et al., 2004).

Even where there is evidence, the effectiveness of a technique is not sufficient to justify its use. We also need to consider the ethical aspects of an approach. To illustrate this point, the practice of using insulin with patients in psychiatric hospitals in the mid-twentieth century could have been argued to be effective in reducing (at least temporarily) the symptoms of depression or a psychotic state, but only through inducing a coma! One important ethical role of research is to investigate the patient/client experience of the therapeutic technique. So with exposure techniques, which deliberately raise a person's level of anxiety, how overwhelming is this for children and young people?

Svensson, Larsson and Ost (2002) examined precisely this question. Fifty-six children and young people, aged 7–17 years, were asked about their experiences of a one-off treatment session for phobias. The session was three hours long and involved exposure to their feared object. The investigators asked the participants how they felt before, during and after treatment. Just over half of the children and young people (52 per cent) said that they had felt nervous prior to treatment. A small number (15 per cent) said specifically that this was anxiety about exposure to the object. Overall, 80 per cent said that they had wanted to take part, and when talking about the therapy itself, most children said they felt in control of the pace of the exposure, with 89 per cent saying the pace had been okay. At the end, 82 per cent said they were satisfied with the outcome of the therapy session, and none expressed that the experience was too stressful for them (Svensson et al., 2002). However, we must bear in mind that this is just one study, and that there may have been some reluctance among children and young people to disclose if the technique was too stressful for them. Indeed, if 82 per cent were satisfied, this leaves 18 per cent who were not, and the study did not account for why this was the case.

Box 7.1   Key studies: What are the effective elements of exposure?

Benito, Conelea, Garcia and Freeman (2012) looked at the moments where exposure was used for 18 children diagnosed with obsessive-compulsive disorder (OCD), aged 4–8 years. They found that the most successful treatments, as measured by reductions on an anxiety scale, contained more of the following elements:

- Therapist discouraging avoidance – e.g. 'keep looking at the sink'
- Externalizing talk – e.g. 'turning these papers away is really going to show OCD who's boss!'
- Exposure comments – rather than 'rescuing' the child from their fears, the therapist or parent makes a statement that may actually increase the child's anxiety, e.g. 'it's possible that something bad might happen to your brother'

Less impact of exposure on the anxiety measure was associated with more:

- Accommodation statements/behaviour – e.g. holding child in their lap
- Unrelated talk – e.g. therapist or parent speaks about something during exposure that is unrelated to the task

An important issue to consider in psychotherapy research is how techniques can work together in progressive and interdependent ways. One study by Peris et al. (2015) of 488 children and young people with anxiety measured the effects of introducing different CBT techniques over time. Relaxation was introduced at week three, cognitive restructuring in the form of altering self-talk was introduced at week five (this involves particularly targeting the undermining ways in which a person may speak to themselves) and graded exposure at week six. The introduction of both cognitive restructuring and exposure was associated with a marked and significant acceleration in the rate of change. However the researchers cautioned that as children had received all three techniques in combination over time, a cumulative effect cannot be ruled out. For example, relaxation may have taken longer to have an effect, or may have helped more in the context of the other two techniques.

Box 7.2   Implications for practice

Graded exposure should be considered for use with children and young people experiencing obsessive-compulsive disorder, specific phobias and post-traumatic stress, bearing in mind their level of tolerance to the exposure tasks.

Cognitive restructuring

Cognitive restructuring involves a range of strategies that are aimed at producing changes to the way a person thinks. The evidence for the relative importance of cognitive restructuring as a technique in CBT with children and young people is mixed. Although far behind in terms of volume of research, this is similar to the picture with adults, which suggests that cognitive techniques are not superior to other techniques and practices (see Cooper, 2008 for a review). In their review of therapies for depression in young people, Kelley, Bickman and Norwood (2010) found that when they compared **meta-analyses** of cognitive to non-cognitive treatments there was no greater efficacy attributed to cognitive techniques, leading the authors to suggest that 'specific alteration of cognitions may not contribute to better outcomes' (2010: 338) with young people.

Two studies have attempted to isolate the effects of cognitive restructuring in particular. For example, Butler, Miezitis, Friedman and Cole (1980) compared the effects of this technique with role play and two other control conditions on children's reports of depression. While the researchers observed both quantitative and qualitative improvements in the role play and cognitive restructuring groups compared to controls, role play showed the largest gains.

Behavioural activation

Behavioural activation looks at activity scheduling and cognitive processes with the aim of encouraging a person to approach activities they have been avoiding, and refocus on rewarding experiences and goals (Veale, 2007). A small study looked at an adapted version of this technique for adolescents experiencing depression. Six young people aged 14–17 attended up to 22 sessions. The study reported significant decreases in depression, and a significant increase in measures of 'hope' among the young people (Ritschel, Ramirez, Jones, & Craighead, 2011). There was no comparison group in this study, although a follow-on study then did look at the effects of this technique in 60 young people compared with a **treatment as usual** group, and the results showed that both conditions in the study produced significant decreases in depression (McCauley et al., 2015). So while the technique of behavioural activation alone may be helpful, there is also evidence that other techniques may be more effective for helping young people with depression (see 'problem solving').

Modelling

There is strong evidence to suggest that modelling techniques can help children and young people to develop less fearful responses to a particular stimulus (whether this be an object or a situation). Modelling involves a parent or therapist demonstrating a non-fearful/relaxed response to the feared stimulus (for example, touching a spider or interacting with a dog in a relaxed manner). Higa-McMillan et al.'s (2015) review suggests that this technique is one of the most potent in reducing anxiety. There is also a lot of evidence to suggest that modelling is one of the most helpful cognitive and behavioural techniques in anger-management therapy with children and young people (Sukhodolsky et al., 2004). This meta-analysis of 40 studies compared the effects of modelling with other techniques such as psychoeducation and exposure for managing anger. Among the 11 CBT techniques compared, modelling, along with homework and feedback techniques, were related to therapeutic outcomes but the other techniques were not.

Assertiveness training

There is some evidence that teaching assertiveness skills in therapy helps children and young people with anxiety. Wehr and Kaufman (1987) compared the effects of assertiveness training with control conditions involving career development training in 96 young people. They found significant differences between the groups, with assertiveness training leading to decreased anxiety. However it is worth considering whether or not this **control group** is an appropriate one, since asking young people to think about their careers could also be viewed as a stressor.

Stress inoculation

Stress inoculation consists of a mixture of other techniques: assertiveness training, progressive muscle relaxation and cognitive restructuring and so, arguably, is a particular combination of techniques rather than one in itself. There is evidence that this can help young people experiencing exam-related anxiety (Kiselica, Baker, Thomas, & Reedy, 1994). However, what was unexpected about the findings of this study was that there was no difference on those students' academic performance. This suggests that anxiety may not be related to exam performance, a counterintuitive finding that may warrant further investigation.

Problem-solving and social skills training

One study comparing techniques in CBT for young people with depression found that those young people who received problem-solving and social skills training were around 2.5 times more likely to benefit from cognitive behavioural therapy than those who did not (Kennard et al., 2009). Other techniques such as cognitive restructuring and behavioural activation were not associated with positive outcomes in the same way; however the young people were not randomly allocated to these techniques, so other factors relating to who was assigned to each group cannot be definitively ruled out. Problem-solving has also been found to be a useful technique in helping children and young people with anger issues (Sukhodolsky et al., 2004).

Psychoeducation

Psychoeducation encompasses a range of educational strategies used to inform people about psychological problems and how to overcome them. It is often used in CBT to educate clients about the cognitive and behavioural principles that underlie their therapy. Psychoeducation has not performed as well as other techniques when compared directly with each other. It has been tested with children and young people with anger issues (Sukhodolsky et al., 2004) as well as in studies dealing with anxiety (Higa-McMillan et al., 2015). However, the results are more promising for a variant of this technique, 'family psychoeducation'. This technique involves family members being taught cognitive behavioural principles in tune with the therapy that a child or young person is receiving. For example, the family may be taught the CBT model of anxiety, including the role of avoidance (or safety behaviours) in maintaining anxiety. There is good support, according to the Higa-McMillan et al. (2015) review, for this technique's efficacy in helping children and young people with anxiety problems.

Box 7.3   Gaps in research

Although cognitive and behavioural techniques have accumulated the largest amount of evidence, more attention needs to be given to techniques other than exposure. For example, it would be useful to know the relative effectiveness of commonly used techniques such as role play and psychoeducation, as well as their acceptability to children and young people, their impact on them and their families, and the best ways that they might be used to enhance therapy.

Humanistic

Empathy, congruence and unconditional positive regard

We saw in Chapter 6 how important 'therapist interpersonal skills' (defined as empathy, warmth and genuineness) are in therapy with children and young people, so it is perhaps not surprising to see the growing evidence supporting the use of humanistic therapies with children and young people, including play therapy and school-based counselling. But when it comes to picking apart the different practices involved in person-centred/ humanistic therapy, there is little at present to go on. Studies demonstrate the importance of the three attitudinal conditions of empathy, unconditional positive regard (UPR) and congruence, but these studies tend to measure these together, with the exception of Green's (1996). This study measured therapist levels of accurate empathy and found a strong association with the amount of engagement of children in their therapy.

One study by Truax, Altman, Wright and Mitchell (1973) looked at the therapeutic process with 15 children with an average age of 9 years. The sessions were with therapists of a mix of orientations, including humanistic, psychodynamic and integrative. The recordings of these sessions were rated by observers, according to the levels of accurate empathy, non-judgemental warmth and genuineness shown by the therapist. The children receiving the therapy were then divided into two groups – those receiving high levels of the three conditions, and those receiving low levels. The researchers then looked at the relationship to outcomes. They found that those receiving high levels showed much greater improvements, and that in fact those receiving low levels actively deteriorated over the course of therapy – their therapy was doing them harm. Due to the sample size, however, it was not possible to disentangle the three therapeutic attitudes from each other to look at the differential effects of these.

Similarly, another study found a 'positive modelling effect' for children who experienced the highest levels of the attitudinal conditions (Siegel, 1972). This meant that those children receiving high levels of empathy, UPR and congruence from their therapists made more insightful and positive statements about themselves by the end of therapy. These findings are further supported by a **qualitative meta-synthesis** on helpful and unhelpful factors for young people receiving counselling in schools. Among the helpful factors cited by young people was the degree to which the counsellor understood them (empathy), and another was the value of talking to someone who was not critical or judgemental (a key aspect of UPR) (Griffiths & Griffiths, 2013).

Box 7.4 Key studies: How are the core conditions of UPR, congruence and empathic understanding experienced and communicated in child-centred play therapy?

A study by Jayne and Ray (2015) aimed to investigate how the attitudinal conditions of client-centred therapy are communicated in play therapy with children aged 4–8 years. This qualitative study involved 12 clients and four therapists. Researchers observed a session with each client through a two-way mirror and interviewed play therapists after the session. They particularly aimed to capture non-verbal as well as verbal communication.

The researchers made the following observations about attitudinal conditions:

- The concept of 'matching' was essential to the experience and communication of empathic understanding of a client. When empathic understanding was realized, play therapists were matching the child's movements, tone, affect, volume and facial expressions.
- Therapist's prior knowledge of a child at different times both aided and blocked empathy. For example, when children acted or played in a manner that was inconsistent or very different from previous sessions, therapists often struggled to stay with the child's immediate experience.
- Therapist incongruence was much easier to identify than congruence.
- When therapists were able to experience a degree of unconditional positive self-regard, this self-acceptance enabled them to demonstrate greater UPR towards the children.
- UPR was communicated consistently through therapists openly receiving children's criticism, corrections and feedback, and through accepting changes or disruptions in the child's play.
- The therapist's experience of congruence, empathy and UPR preceded and enabled the expression of these attitudes towards the child. When this was done using specific skills such as tracking, reflections, leaning towards a child or turning, without the internal experience of these attitudes, this was insufficient as a communication of the core conditions to the client.

Box 7.5   Implications for practice

It is important in therapy to display accurate empathic understanding to children and young people.

Psychodynamic

Interpretation

This technique is typically found to be used to a greater degree in the later phases of treatment (Goodman, 2015; Trowell, Rhode, Miles, & Sherwood, 2003), and refers to the comments a therapist makes regarding a patient's (verbal or non-verbal) communication, that go beyond what the patient has consciously acknowledged. While the technique is a core component of psychodynamic practice, and some interesting research has been done with adults (e.g. Høglend et al., 2008), its effectiveness with young people has not yet been assessed in meta-analytic studies. However, Fonagy and Moran's (1990) study correlating interpretations of unconscious conflict in therapy sessions and improvements in control of brittle diabetes is a noteworthy example of research that does evaluate the efficacy of interpretation against biochemical outcome measures. This study showed that the interpretation of unconscious conflict and anxieties around patients' diabetic regimens predicted improvements in diabetic management. The findings suggest that this technique mitigates self-destructive behaviours and is an effective method to restore metabolic equilibrium in young people with this condition.

A more recent study by Luzzi, Bardi, Ramos and Slapak (2015), examining types of interpretations and responses across child psychoanalytic therapy, concludes that interpretation is an effective technique when dealing with expressions of anxiety in children, and that both transference and extra-transference interpretations correlate with the children's progress in symbolic processes and self-control. However, Luzzi, Bardi, Ramos and Slapak's (2015) results are only preliminary due to a small sample size and lack of control group. See Kennedy and Midgley (2007) for a comprehensive review of child, adolescent and parent–infant psychotherapy process studies and related measures.

Transference interpretations

The most commonly studied form of interpretations in child and adult research are transference interpretations, by which is meant statements made by the therapist referring to the relationship between the patient and therapist, with a particular focus on how the patient feels towards the therapist or therapeutic setting. A follow-up study of former child patients specifically examines what attitudes patients had towards being in therapy and what they remembered as adults of the therapy and their therapist (Midgley & Target, 2005). Highlighting the prominence former patients placed on the interpersonal qualities of the relationship, namely the therapist as a sympathetic and non-judgemental listener, the study also reported on the fact that some former patients appeared to value significant interpretations made by the therapist that helped develop their self-understanding, even decades after the event.

An important dimension of transference interpretations is not only the initial interpretation by the therapist but the reaction from the patient, as well as then the therapist's response to this – that which has been called in adult research, the 'third interpretative turn' (Perakyla, 2010). Della Rosa (2016) investigates these elaborations between patient and therapist of transference interpretations in four cases of short-term (28 sessions) psychoanalytic therapy with depressed adolescents. The results show that transference tended not to be explicitly discussed between therapist and patient, but rather, when it was done, it was through the use of metaphor, to carry the topic over into a new representative form.

A complementary approach to the study of conversational details that is potentially relevant for this line of research may be the qualitative studies mapping the moment-by-moment of interactions via microanalysis methods (Harrison, 2014; Leudar, Sharrock, Truckle, Colombino, Hayes, & Booth, 2008), which can pick up on subtleties such as the prosody, word choice and timing, and how they coalesce to establish therapeutic occasions.

Box 7.6   Key studies: What are transference interpretations about?

Topics that therapists made the focus of their transference interpretations with adolescents in Della Rosa's (2016) study were categorized into four themes:

1. Negative or conflicting feelings towards the therapist
2. Issues of dependency relating to resistance or attachment to the therapist
3. The wish for more sessions and fears of rejection
4. Difficulty in expressing feelings towards the therapist

The author notes that the themes of the interpretations tended to centre on issues of separation such as dependency and infantile needs. They noted a corresponding lack of other central aspects of adolescent psychodynamic theory, such as sexuality. It would be of interest to know whether this concentration of themes is particular to these cases, their age group, or particular diagnoses.

Dream interpretations

Reports of dream interpretation are usually limited to clinical case studies (Adamo, 2012; Barrett, 2016), however, a review by Lempen and Midgley (2006) reports that references to dream analysis in child therapy have declined in the clinical literature over the last 50 years. Empirical research mirrors this, with the majority of child psychotherapists in the study by Lempen and Midgley (2006) reporting that they do not actively suggest talking about dreams to children in therapy. The study also interviewed four child therapists in depth about their practice of interpreting dreams, and found that a shift away from interpretations of dreams and unconscious meaning was understood to be the result of a greater focus on transference interpretations and working with the relationship in the here-and-now. The results of the study show that there was significant disagreement on techniques of working with dreams in child therapy – for example, whether to consider it a form of free association relating to the session or whether interpreting the dream in terms of the relationship with the therapist was 'potentially intrusive' (2006: 243). However, all participants agreed on the importance of the play that followed children's reports of dreams, as this was viewed as a way of observing the child's own associations and a way of elaborating on the meaning of the dream.

Box 7.7 Implications for practice

When using interpretation techniques with children and adolescents, therapists should pay particular attention to their elaboration via play or metaphor.

Mirroring

One study has shown mirroring techniques to be in popular use with young people receiving psychoanalytic therapy for depression. The study by Trowell et al. (2003) with 10–14 year olds found that mirroring techniques – a therapist's reflections of the client's experience and descriptions of how the client might feel (see communications of empathy outlined in Chapter 6) – were used by therapists as much as interpretation. This study also shed light on what therapists considered the relevant elements of their sessions. In comparing the audio-recordings of the sessions with the therapists' process notes, Trowell et al. (2003) found that non-interpretative interventions, such as mirroring, clarifications or questioning, tended to be edited or compressed in process notes, but interpretations were accurately reflected. An implication of this is that these non-interpretative techniques would be less reported in clinical cases and supervision, and may as a consequence be underemphasized in psychodynamic theory. This study raises questions about what methods therapists are using in the session to bring about therapeutic processes. And why might they be doing things differently to 'the model' – for example, do they have to be more flexible with younger people?

Countertransference

Therapists' use of their own countertransference, often supported by supervision, is considered an important practice in psychodynamic therapy. Few studies have directly examined the nature of this practice in detail. However, a paper published by Ulberg et al. (2013) shows that a therapist's countertransference feelings, specifically ones described as 'confident' (i.e. warm and playful feelings), are associated with strong therapeutic alliances.

A number of studies have been carried out illustrating how countertransference patterns and therapy processes are interwoven (Goodman & Mavrides, 2010; Ruzansky 2007). Goodman's (2015) findings, making use of the Child Psychotherapy Q-Set (CPQ, Schneider & Jones, 2004), show how different interaction structures are formed between a therapist and a child in a study where one child was treated by two different therapists. This indicates that therapist-specific and dyad-specific effects may be relevant to understanding why an effective treatment may work with one dyad and not with another. While not focused directly on techniques, the CPQ – and its equivalent for adolescents, the Adolescent Psychotherapy Q-Set (Bychkova, Hillman, Midgley, & Schneider, 2011) – is a potentially relevant tool. In practice, effective therapy is never going to be based on the use of individual techniques used in isolation but on how a therapist's technique changes across the course of a therapy, partly in response to changes in how a child engages and the kind of interaction structures that develop between therapist and child. Studies that explore the interaction of different techniques and patterns are a promising area of research to explore what factors contribute to therapeutic change, beyond the study of individual 'techniques'.

Arts and play

Play

Psychoanalysis began the tradition of using play to help children work through their psychological difficulties by understanding play as a form of symbolic communication that represents psychological states. Whether it is a technique or better described as a therapeutic medium, the use of play with children in therapy is now very well supported, both in humanistic and filial play therapy, which involves training parents to use therapeutic play with their children (Bratton, Ray, Rhine, & Jones, 2005). The power of this technique perhaps lies partly in the ability of play to transcend language and so is an important means of symbolization for those with limited access to language.

Music

Findings suggest that the use of music in therapy with children and adolescents may be highly beneficial, with most research carried out in the context of music therapy (Gold, Voracek, & Wigram, 2004). One research study has broken down music therapy into some component techniques in order to determine the effects of these (Gold, Wigram, & Voracek, 2007). It compared the following commonly used techniques with 77 children aged 4–19:

- Improvisation – unstructured, free expression through music
- Pre-composed music – structured playing of a pre-written song
- Verbal reflection – discussion of topics experienced and discovered through the music
- Use of other media and play activities – non-musical activities, often used with children who are not ready to engage with music
- Receptive work – listening to music and reflecting on this.

The study found most benefits from the use of improvisation and verbal reflection. The use of other media and play was associated with an absence of improvement. However, the authors of this study cautioned that this latter technique may be confounded with client 'motivation to change' (see Chapter 6) – as this technique is more often used with clients who are not yet ready to engage with music (Gold et al., 2007).

Art

There is very little research that compares the use of art in therapy with children and young people to not using this medium. At present there is no evidence to suggest that therapies using art are superior or inferior to those that rely on the traditional format of talking (Reynolds, Nabors, & Quinlan, 2000). This review of 17 studies included five **randomized controlled trials** – three of which showed benefits in the art therapy group relative to the control group and two showing no significant differences.

Some of the benefits that have been highlighted in qualitative and quantitative research on the use of art in therapy with children include:

- Children are better able to express their emotions
- Leading to a greater ability to cope with feelings
- Increases in self-esteem
- Reduction in trauma-based symptoms
- Greater emotional connection and comfort with physical proximity for toddlers with their caregivers (see Slayton, D'Archer, & Kaplan, 2010, for a review).

Drama

There is a small amount of evidence pointing towards the helpfulness of using drama as a technique in group therapy with young people. For example, this has been tested with children with social anxiety (Dadsetan, Anari, & Sedghpour, 2008), young refugees experiencing trauma (Rousseau et al., 2007) and girls who had been sexually abused

(MacKay, Gold, & Gold, 1987). All three studies reported significant differences in measures of psychological problems after the drama therapy. One paper explained the effectiveness of this technique as providing 'a metaphorical space where trauma and loss can be expressed and transformed' (Rousseau et al., 2007: 463). However only one of the studies (Dadsetan, Anari, & Sedghpour, 2008) used a **randomized controlled trial** design, so more research is needed to confirm the effectiveness of the use of drama in therapy with children and young people in a range of contexts.

Box 7.8   Implications for practice

Creative processes may be alternative methods for exploring and expressing emotions, especially when language is limited.

Narrative

Cultural storytelling

Cultural storytelling is a narrative-based technique that involves the telling of stories in a therapeutic group with the use of culturally appropriate stimuli such as pictures and cartoons and through the use of psychodrama. This method has been demonstrated to be effective in helping young people with anxiety problems, with the evidence coming from one study with 90 children and young people aged 9–13, in the US and of Hispanic heritage. Half of the group were randomized to a 'cultural storytelling' condition of eight weekly sessions of 90 minutes in groups. The main materials were a collection of pictures that depicted scenes relevant to Hispanic culture including typical neighbourhoods, foods and gender roles. The artist had previously researched relevant elements for inclusion through consultation with 'cultural experts' (Costantino, Malgady, & Rogler, 1994: 16). Each session involved the following steps:

1. The participants were given a pre-selected series of pictures and were asked to produce a story about what was happening in these scenes.
2. They were then asked to share their personal experiences in relation to the pictures with the therapist who 'verbally reinforced themes that were . . . adaptive. . . . Maladaptive themes were referred to the group to discuss alternative, more adaptive resolutions of personal conflict' (1994: 16).
3. Psychodrama was used to perform the scenes in the original story and then a videotape was played back to them and discussed.

The aim of the intervention was to help the young people develop more adaptive patterns of thinking and behaving. The control group instead watched age-appropriate films (e.g. *Pinocchio* and *Star Wars*) that were not culturally tailored, and discussed them afterwards with the therapist. They also drew the characters that they liked, and dramatized the themes or actions of their favourite characters in the films. This condition was structured to be as similar as possible to the cultural storytelling condition.

The use of cultural storytelling was found to be more effective in reducing anxiety, fear and conduct problems in the children and young people than the control condition, accounting for 4 per cent of the **variance** in clinical outcomes, which is a d of 0.41, in other words a small to medium effect (Costantino et al., 1994). The authors speculated whether cultural sensitivity is therapeutic in itself, or whether it indirectly enabled the effects of 'modelling' – namely learning from the successful characters in the stories – to happen.

Box 7.9   Implications for practice

Cultural storytelling may be a relevant intervention for young people experiencing anxiety problems who live in communities in which they are ethnic minorities.

General

Giving advice and making suggestions

A consistent finding in **qualitative research** with young people about what they found helpful about therapy includes the advice given by a counsellor or therapist. In a collection of studies looking at the effects of school-based counselling, Griffiths and Griffiths (2013) found that young people not only highlighted the space to talk and be listened to non-judgementally, but also the advice and suggestions given by the counsellors (who were all person-centred in orientation). This finding has also been noted by Karver, Handelsman, Fields, Bickman and Bickman's (2006) meta-analysis, which cites 'therapist direct influencing skills' as having a strong association to outcomes.

Exactly what this involves, however, is in need of illumination through qualitative research. Cooper's (2004) study, for example, indicates that how this advice is provided is crucial – and that young people find advice more helpful when it has the character of 'possibilities' and 'suggestions' rather than 'instructions and directives' (Cooper, 2004). Given that the way young people are given advice seems an important component of effective therapy, more research is clearly needed into how best this can be done.

Goals

Setting mutually agreed goals in therapy with adults has been associated with good clinical outcomes, and client motivation and engagement (see Cooper, 2008). There are no equivalent studies with children and young people that compare setting goals with not setting goals for therapy, but there has been research showing that, firstly, setting goals in therapy is meaningful to children and young people, and they can come up with their own goals, if not initially, then over time (McCrea, 2014). However goal-setting in the context of therapy with children is complex. For example, one study involving 315 children and adolescents, aged 7–17, their parents and their therapists, noted a significant lack of agreement between the three parties on what the target problems in therapy should be (Hawley & Weisz, 2003). The authors found that only 23.2 per cent of child–therapist–parent triads could agree on any target problems, although agreement on externalizing problems was greater than other kinds of problems, changing aggressive behaviour, in particular, achieving the most achievement as a goal. Moreover, therapists were much more likely to agree with parents' goals than children's goals, with 76.3 per cent agreeing with at least one parent goal, and 52 per cent with at least one child goal (Hawley & Weisz, 2003).

Another study examined the themes of goals that were being set by children and parents in therapy. The authors found that children tended to set goals that were more related to their personal growth and dealing with specific problems, while parents' goals focused on more general strategies to help their child (for example, how to achieve a better bedtime routine), and managing their behaviour (Jacob, Murphy, Fugard, Nolas, & Law, 2016). For more on goals, see Box 7.10.

Box 7.10   Key studies: Whose goals are they anyway?

Edbrooke-Childs, Jacob, Law, Deighton and Wolpert (2015) examined the data from 137 children from 14 different child and adolescent mental health services (CAMHS) in the UK. They found that of these goals:

- 42 per cent were recorded as jointly agreed between the child, parents and therapist
- 25 per cent were set by the child only
- 13 per cent by the parent
- 2 per cent by the therapist

This suggests a picture of more goal agreement than the earlier study by Hawley and Weisz (2003). However, these studies were in different service contexts (US vs UK) and the data collected for the two studies were 10–15 years apart in time. Perhaps the process of goal-setting has become more collaborative over time?

Taken together then, these findings confirm the experience of many therapists that children and their parents arrive at therapy with different priorities and expectations for what therapy will help with. It highlights the importance of the process of setting goals – for example, is achieving agreement on all goals necessary? How much agreement is enough agreement? How does the role power of the therapist and parent influence goal-setting with children and young people? Clearly, more research is needed into the effects of jointly agreed versus individual goals on how beneficial the process is overall, and into how this process is best facilitated by therapists.

Manuals

Manuals in this context are written documents that outline the procedures and methods for how to deliver a therapy. The use of manuals in therapy is controversial – on the one hand, they have the potential to offer guidance to therapists, and standardization of the therapy that is offered; on the other hand, some therapists are concerned that they may stifle the creativity needed to respond to a child's unique and changing needs. One study has shown that such concerns tend to reduce once therapists have actually experienced using a treatment manual (Henton & Midgley, 2012), but what does the evidence say about the effect of manuals on the therapeutic alliance, which some have argued may in particular be compromised by the use of manuals? This is an important question given research findings that point towards the importance of flexibility in forming strong alliances with children and young people (Hudson et al., 2014; Zack, Castonguay, & Boswell, 2007). Two studies have tested this, and demonstrated that the use of manuals in fact does not seem to undermine the therapeutic alliance with children and young people (Langer, McLeod, & Weisz, 2011; McLeod et al., 2016). In one study, half of the young people receiving therapy for anxiety and depression took part in CBT from therapists who were guided by a manual. The other half worked with therapists instructed to 'employ the therapeutic procedures they used regularly and believed to be effective' (Langer et al., 2011: 428). Results indicated that the use of manuals was associated with a stronger alliance early in therapy, which declined over time. Clients in the non-manualized group reported the opposite trend, with alliance increasing over the course of therapy. There was no difference in the overall strength of the alliance between the two groups when the whole course of therapy was examined. The authors suggested that these curious findings may be due to the manual-guided therapies offering a clear structure and agenda at the beginning of therapy, helping those clients who did not know what to expect from therapy (see Chapter 6 on client expectations). Perhaps the alliance then declines in the manualized therapies due to lower levels of flexibility that these therapies may afford?

Some caution is needed however in interpreting the scope of these findings. The comparison condition of 'no manual' may not reflect the non-manualized therapies that are practised in normal clinical practice conditions. For example, many practitioners who do not use manuals may be guided by other things such as a body of theory, their supervisor and feedback from clients. There is also little information about how detailed and prescriptive the manuals were as guides to practice. We also saw in Chapter 6 how one study has reported that 'rigid adherence' to **treatment protocols** does seem to undermine the alliance (Zack et al., 2007). Clearly, further research in this area is needed in order to determine how helpful manuals are in work with children and young people, and how detailed these should be.

Mindfulness

Mindfulness is an increasingly popular approach in therapeutic work with adults, and initial evidence suggests that there are benefits of using mindfulness techniques with children and adolescents too. There are now a handful of studies indicating that mindfulness and meditation techniques may not only help children and young people with feelings of anxiety (Semple, Lee, Rosa, & Miller, 2010; Wall, 2005), but also with attention and self-control problems (Bögels, Hoogstad, van Dun, de Schutter, & Restifo, 2008).

This area of research is interesting not only due to the therapeutic techniques involved but because it demonstrates the beginning stages of how evidence for a therapeutic technique may accumulate and evolve. An early study showed the benefits of teaching meditation to schoolchildren on their ability to concentrate in distracting environments (Linden, 1973). This was not psychotherapy research per se, but it showed that these techniques could be taught successfully to children. More recently, a small-scale study examined the use of a mindfulness group therapy based in a school, with 7 and 8 year olds. Six sessions of 45 minutes took place weekly with five children. This study showed that not only did children of this age engage and enjoy the exercises, but that all showed improvements either in self-reported anxiety, or in their academic performance, by the end of the six weeks. This study was particularly well reported because it described in some detail exactly what these techniques involved, and how the different children responded to them (see Semple, Reid, & Miller, 2005).

Having established the 'feasibility' and acceptability to children (in the US) of mindfulness techniques, Semple et al. (2010) ran a randomized controlled trial involving 25 children, aged 9–13 years. All of these children had been referred because they were having problems with reading at school. Half of the group received mindfulness-based cognitive therapy, and these were compared to a **wait-list control group**. The researchers observed significant improvements in attention-related problems, and some changes in anxiety and behavioural problems (Semple et al., 2010).

There is evidence too that involving parents in mindfulness training is also therapeutically beneficial. In one study with 14 young people diagnosed with ADHD and other attention and conduct problems, young people received mindfulness training as a group and parents were offered 'mindful parent training' in parallel (Bögels et al., 2008). By the end of the eight-week training and at an eight-week follow-up, the young people reported substantial gains in many areas of their lives, including their ability to concentrate. Parents also reported significant improvements in their children, including their ability to exercise self-control and attunement to others. Parents also improved in working towards their own goals (Bögels et al., 2008).

Mindfulness therapies have not yet been compared with non-mindfulness therapies – meaning that we cannot be absolutely sure that the mindfulness techniques alone are accounting for the changes observed and that some other factor – for example, being in a supportive group with others – is not more important. However the evidence is looking promising for using mindfulness as a therapeutic technique with children and their parents.

Box 7.11   Implications for practice

Mindfulness is a helpful practice to consider for young people with concentration and self-control problems, as well as for their parents.

Relaxation

There is some evidence to suggest that the use of relaxation techniques – such as progressive muscle relaxation and breathing exercises – can help children and young people experiencing anxiety or depression. In a study by Reynolds and Coats (1986) relaxation was compared to CBT (containing components such as those techniques included above). Relaxation was just as helpful in relieving depression, and also reduced reports of anxiety. In a qualitative study of counselling in schools, relaxation exercises were cited (spontaneously) by young people as a beneficial factor in the humanistic therapy they received (Cooper, 2004).

Self-hypnosis

Teaching self-hypnosis to children and young people has good evidence of effectiveness in reducing feelings of anxiety, according to a recent review (Higa-McMillan et al., 2015). In one study, Stanton (1994) measured the effects of a self-hypnosis technique for young people aged 12–15. Forty students were randomly allocated to either the self-hypnosis group or a control group. The self-hypnosis group learned a technique in two sessions of 50 minutes each. There was a significant reduction on measures of 'test anxiety' in comparison to the control group and this was maintained even after six months.

Box 7.12   Key studies: Practices of self-disclosure with young people

There is not yet any empirical work linking therapist self-disclosure of personal information to outcomes with children and young people, but one interesting study has recently looked at how and why therapists self-disclose with young people. In this study the researcher interviewed 12 therapists working with clients aged 14–18 years about the ways they use self-disclosure in their work and their motivations for doing so (Smith, 2010).

The researcher found that all participants gave the matter significant forethought before disclosing something about themselves. The following kinds of things were disclosed:

- previous life experiences;
- techniques and strategies used for dealing with problems;
- reactions to clients or the therapeutic process.

The therapists' motivations for disclosure included:

- normalizing the young person's struggles;
- to model or teach skills;
- to build or strengthen the therapeutic relationship;
- to help a client to gain insight into themselves;
- to get therapy 'unstuck'.

The author found that therapists who self-disclosed about the here-and-now relationship with the young person did so exclusively in order to help move the therapeutic process out of what they perceived as a stuck phase. Furthermore, the type of self-disclosure used was dependent on the age of the young person – with therapists saying that they tended to use more concrete, skills-based/modelling disclosures with younger children or children functioning at a lower developmental level and, with adolescents, they tended to use a wider variety of self-disclosure (including sharing past experiences and commenting on the here-and-now relationship).

Session-by-session feedback

There is preliminary evidence that the use of session-by-session feedback – where a child/young person is asked to fill out a brief questionnaire each session indicating their views on the therapy, and the therapist uses this feedback to tailor the therapy – may have a positive association with therapeutic change with children. The evidence comes from just one study so far, which was a **pre-post design**. This was with 288 children aged 7–11 who were receiving school-based counselling of a range of modalities (CBT, narrative, person-centred, play therapy). The use of session-by-session feedback was associated with a large effect on a range of outcome measures, although no comparison group was used (Cooper, Stewart, Sparks, & Bunting, 2013).

Touch

Research in adult therapies suggests that, under certain conditions, physical contact with a therapist can be a good experience for clients. For example, this was experienced as helpful or unhelpful depending on factors such as: whether the client felt in control, the timing of the touch, and whether this was felt to be due to the client's needs, rather than the therapist's needs. Positive consequences have been reported as feeling a sense of care and acceptance from a therapist; but negative consequences include that the client may perceive the therapist as vulnerable and in need of looking after, and thus inhibit their needs in relation to the therapist (see Cooper, 2008, for a full discussion). In all circumstances, the type of touch that has been investigated is of course non-sexual in nature – sexual contact with clients of all ages is prohibited by all professional codes of ethics.

When working with children and young people, our awareness of power dynamics in therapy should be even more acute – and this makes touch as a 'technique' a very delicate area. Some organizations may preclude this outright in their policies. But even in these situations, some circumstances may force the issue onto a therapist; for example if a child is climbing and about to fall, or perhaps spontaneously grabs a therapist's leg as they leave their session. These situations are not so much about touch as an intentional action but as a response to an unfolding situation.

Unfortunately, there is next to nothing in terms of empirical work in this area to support and guide practice (there is, however, an excellent theoretical paper by McNeil-Haber, 2004). One older study showed that 'tactile and verbal reinforcement' was more effective in helping 9–11 year old boys to concentrate in class than 'verbal reinforcement alone' (Clements & Tracey, 1977, as cited in McNeil-Haber, 2004). However, there are no equivalent studies with children that examine their experiences of touch in therapy.

Box 7.13   Gaps in research

There is a need for evidence on the use of touch in therapy with children and young people. This should include more understanding of the circumstances in which this occurs, the conditions in which this might be helpful, and why, and the conditions in which this might be unhelpful, and why. This research should gather the experiences of children and young people, their therapists, and their caregivers and families.

Working with strengths

There is evidence that giving attention to the strengths of children and young people is an effective way of helping them, although most of this evidence does not examine psychotherapy only, but other helping settings such as social work (Brownlee et al., 2013). One study did show that a strengths focus can be very successful in psychotherapy with young people (Cox, 2006). This found that those therapists with a stronger 'strengths orientation' were achieving better outcomes with children and young people. In this study, therapists were rated by observers as to how much attention to strengths they were giving in their sessions with young people. Those with a stronger 'strengths orientation' were showing better therapeutic outcomes with young people.

Box 7.14 Key studies: Use of strengths in therapy for substance abuse

Harris, Brazeau, Clarkson, Brownlee and Rawana (2012) used a qualitative approach to investigate young people's experiences of a strengths-based inpatient therapy for substance use. This was interesting as it reported on what types of strengths were important for these young people to become aware of in themselves and which ones were helping them to overcome their difficulties.

The study consisted of 52 interviews taken with young people aged 15–18 years after taking part in a five-week residential programme. This could be regarded therefore as a fairly intensive course of therapy. In the interviews, young people were asked a range of questions about their experiences of the programme. One question – 'what information did you receive in treatment that was most helpful to you?' – yielded very interesting answers. The young people had received three broad interventions – CBT, relapse prevention and strengths-based – and they highlighted the strengths-based activities consistently above the other techniques.

The particular strengths that they identified as becoming aware of, and developing in therapy, largely related to their interpersonal skills, including:

- their sense of humour;
- ability to act as a leader;
- ability to draw on positive peer relationships;
- ability to ask others for support.

The last skill was identified as a major area that young people had struggled with in the past and felt more confident with after therapy. They also mentioned the usefulness of setting and accomplishing goals, and that having goals for the future was in fact a new thing for them.

Other themes from the interviews included the importance of being brave and showing resilience to deal with life problems and difficult emotions without using drugs.

The authors noted how popular the strengths-based techniques seemed to be with these young people and how readily they adopted them. Perhaps this focus was refreshing – many of the young people interviewed said that they were not used to thinking of themselves as having any strengths, and were much more used to having conversations about where they were going wrong in their lives.

Conclusion

We would love to conclude this chapter with some nice snappy headlines about the best practices and techniques in therapy with children and young people. However, we fear we would be misrepresenting the truth. This is because the current size of the evidence base makes it difficult to reliably produce definitive statements about the 'best' techniques and practices to use with children and young people. The research in its current state is sparse and is often clustered around particular diagnoses such as anxiety, depression and substance misuse. It is also largely focused on cognitive and behavioural techniques.

There are also some issues – that intersect with the theories and aims of different practices – that mean that making direct comparisons is hard. In terms of outcomes and their measurement, are all techniques and practices aiming to produce the same kind of change? And when it comes to remit, are some specific techniques targeted at very specific symptoms, and other practices designed to engage with the 'messier' problems of life?

However, with these caveats in mind, we will summarize some tentative findings.

Summary of key findings

- A range of techniques and practices from different schools of therapy have been shown to have a helpful impact in work with children and young people. This evidence comes from a variety of sources: randomized controlled trials, pre-post designs, qualitative feedback from clients and studies of therapy sessions.
- Cognitive and behavioural techniques, particularly for anxiety, have received the most research attention. There is now firm research supporting the use of exposure as a technique for anxiety.
- There is evidence in support of using modelling for helping children and young people with anxiety and anger issues, and problem-solving to help with depression.
- Humanistic practices – such as empathy, congruence and unconditional positive regard – have been packaged in different ways in research in child and adolescent therapies. They have been associated with therapeutic personality change and good therapeutic relationships/alliances in these various packages.
- Psychodynamic research highlights both the therapist's use of techniques as well as the patient's response to them, suggesting that interaction structures are relevant to understanding how therapeutic methods work.
- There is some evidence to support the use of methods other than talking in therapy with children and young people, including play, art, music and drama.
- There is initial evidence showing the effects of several techniques and practices that do not belong to just a single therapy approach.
- These include that young people consistently say that they like some advice and suggestions from their therapists – but that the way that this is done is important.
- Engaging with the strengths that young people have, as well as their problems, is associated with good outcomes and client engagement.

Recommended reading

Cooper, M. (2008). Technique and practice factors. In M. Cooper, *Essential research findings in counselling and psychotherapy: The facts are friendly*. London: Sage. This is an accessible summary of the research findings about techniques and practices in therapies with adults.

Lepper, G., & Riding, N. (2006). *Researching the psychotherapy process: a practical guide to transcript-based methods*. Palgrave Macmillan. Primarily a guide to how to conduct psychotherapy process research, but includes many interesting examples of studies, mostly from the field of adult psychotherapy.

Shirk, S. R., & Russell, R. L. (1996). *Change processes in child psychotherapy: Revitalizing treatment and research*. New York: Guilford Press. Although slightly out of date, this book provides a valuable history of researchers' attempts to investigate the therapy process with children and young people.

Questions for reflection

- What techniques and practices do you use regularly with children/young people, and why do you use these? Were you trained to use these techniques? Does the theory you use tell you to? Have you learnt something about using these through your experience?
- What kind of evidence would you need to see to change your mind about your current practices? What would convince you to try a new technique or practice, or to change something you are already doing?
- This chapter has presented some individual studies that have used different research methods. Which studies did you find most helpful or convincing, and why?

References

Adamo, S. M. G. (2012). The aesthetic experience in the process of recovery from autistic states. *Journal of Child Psychotherapy*, 38, 61–77.

Barrett, D. (2016). Dream weaver/dream catcher: The older child and analyst at work. *Psychoanalytic Inquiry*, 36, 242–254.

Benito, K. G., Conelea, C., Garcia, A. M., & Freeman, J. B. (2012). CBT specific process in exposure-based treatments: Initial examination in a pediatric OCD sample. *Journal of Obsessive-Compulsive and Related Disorders*, 1, 77–84.

Bögels, S., Hoogstad, B., van Dun, L., de Schutter, S., & Restifo, K. (2008). Mindfulness training for adolescents with externalizing disorders and their parents. *Behavioural and Cognitive Psychotherapy*, 36, 193–209.

Bratton, S. C., Ray, D., Rhine, T., & Jones, L. (2005). The efficacy of play therapy with children: A meta-analytic review of treatment outcomes. *Professional Psychology: Research and Practice*, 36, 376–390.

Brownlee, K., Rawana, J., Franks, J., Harper, J., Bajwa, J., O'Brien, E., & Clarkson, A. (2013). A systematic review of strengths and resilience outcome literature relevant to children and adolescents. *Child and Adolescent Social Work Journal*, 30, 435–459.

Butler, L., Miezitis, S., Friedman, R., & Cole, E. (1980). The effect of two school-based intervention programs on depressive symptoms in preadolescents. *American Education Research Journal*, 17, 111–119.

Bychkova, T., Hillman, S., Midgley, N., & Schneider, C. (2011). The psychotherapy process with adolescents: Preliminary comparisons between different therapeutic modalities using the Adolescent Psychotherapy Q-Set. *Journal of Child Psychotherapy*, 37, 327–348.

Clements, J. E., & Tracy, D. B. (1977). Effects of touch and verbal reinforcement on the classroom behavior of emotionally disturbed boys. *Exceptional Children*, 43, 453–454.

Cohen, J. A., Berliner, L., & Mannarino, A. P. (2000). Treatment of traumatized children: A review and synthesis. *Journal of Trauma, Violence and Abuse*, 1, 29–46.

Costantino, G., Malgady, R. G., & Rogler, L. H. (1994). Storytelling through pictures: Culturally sensitive psychotherapy for Hispanic children and adolescents. *Journal of Clinical Child Psychology*, 23, 13–20.

Cooper, M. (2004). Towards a relationally-orientated approach to therapy: Empirical support and analysis. *British Journal of Guidance and Counselling*, 32, 451–460.

Cooper, M. (2008). *Essential research findings in counselling and psychotherapy: The facts are friendly.* London: Sage.

Cooper, M., Stewart, D., Sparks, J., & Bunting, L. (2013). School-based counseling using systematic feedback: A cohort study evaluating outcomes and predictors of change. *Psychotherapy Research*, 23, 474–488.

Cox, K. F. (2006). Investigating the impact of strength-based assessment on youth with emotional or behavioral disorders. *Journal of Child and Family Studies*, 15, 287–301.

Dadsetan, P., Anari, A., & Sedghpour, B. S. (2008). Social anxiety disorders and drama-therapy. *Journal of Iranian Psychologists*, 4, 115–123.

Della Rosa, E. (2016). An exploration of transference interpretations in short term psychoanalytic psychotherapy with adolescents suffering from depression. Unpublished doctoral dissertation, Tavistock NHS Trust and University of East London.

Edbrooke-Childs, J., Jacob, J., Law, D., Deighton, J., & Wolpert, M. (2015). Interpreting standardized and idiographic outcome measures in CAMHS: What does change mean and how does it relate to functioning and experience? *Child and Adolescent Mental Health*, 20, 142–148.

Fonagy, P., & Moran, G. S. (1990). Studies of the efficacy of child psychoanalysis. *Journal of Consulting and Clinical Psychology*, 58, 684–695.

Gold, C., Voracek, M., & Wigram, T. (2004). Effects of music therapy for children and adolescents with psychopathology: A meta-analysis. *Journal of Child Psychology and Psychiatry*, 45, 1054–1063.

Gold, C., Wigram, T., & Voracek, M. (2007). Predictors of change in music therapy with children and adolescents: The role of therapeutic techniques. *Psychology and Psychotherapy*, 80, 577–589.

Goodman, G. (2015). Interaction structures between a child and two therapists in the psychodynamic treatment of a child with borderline personality disorders. *Journal of Child Psychotherapy*, 41, 141–161.

Goodman, G., & Mavrides, L. (2010). Countertransference, process, and outcome in psychodynamic child psychotherapy. Paper presented at the meeting of the Society for Psychotherapy Research, Asilomar, CA.

Green, J. M. (1996). Engagement and empathy: A pilot study of the therapeutic alliance in outpatient child psychiatry. *Child Psychology and Psychiatry Review*, 1, 130–138.

Griffiths, L., & Griffiths, C. (2013). Unconditional positive self-regard (UPSR) and self-compassion, the internal consistency and convergent/divergent validity of Patterson & Joseph's UPSR scale. *Open Journal of Medical Psychology*, 2, 168–174.

Harris, N., Brazeau, J. N., Clarkson, A., Brownlee, K., & Rawana, E. (2012). Adolescents' experiences of a strengths-based treatment program for substance abuse. *Journal of Psychoactive Drugs*, 44, 390–397.

Harrison, A. (2014). The sandwich model: The 'music and dance' of therapeutic action. *International Journal of Psychoanalysis*, 95, 313–340.

Hawley, K. M., & Weisz, J. R. (2003). Child, parent, and therapist (dis)agreement on target problems in outpatient therapy: The therapist's dilemma and its implications. *Journal of Consulting and Clinical Psychology*, 71, 62–70.

Henton, I., & Midgley, N. (2012). 'A path in the woods': A study of child psychotherapists' participation in a large randomised controlled trial. *Counselling and Psychotherapy Research*, 12, 204–213.

Higa-McMillan, C. K., Francis, S. E., Rith-Najarian, L., & Chorpita, B. F. (2015). Evidence base update: 50 years of research on treatment for child and adolescent anxiety. *Journal of Clinical Child and Adolescent Psychology*, 45, 91–113.

Høglend, P., Bøgwald, K. P., Amlo, S., Marble, A., Ulberg, R., Sjaastad, M., Sørbye, Ø., Heyerdahl, O., & Johansson, P. (2008). Transference interpretations in dynamic psychotherapy: Do they really yield sustained effects? *American Journal of Psychiatry*, 165, 763–771.

Hudson, J. L., Kendall, P. C., Chu, B. C., Gosch, E., Martin, E., Taylor, A., & Knight, A. (2014). Child involvement, alliance, and therapist flexibility: Process variables in cognitive-behavioural therapy for anxiety disorders in childhood. *Behaviour Research and Therapy*, 52, 1–8.

Jacob, J., Murphy, S., Fugard, A. J. B., Nolas, M., & Law, D. (2016). What kind of goals do children and young people set for themselves in therapy? Developing a goals framework using CORC data. *Clinical Child and Family Psychology Review*, 1, 8–18.

Jayne, K. M., & Ray, D. C. (2015). Therapist-provided conditions in child-centered play therapy. *Journal of Humanistic Counseling*, 54, 86–103.

Karver, M. S., Handelsman, J. B., Fields, S., Bickman, L., & Bickman, L. (2006). Meta-analysis of therapeutic relationship variables in youth and family therapy: The evidence for different relationship variables in the child and adolescent treatment outcome literature. *Clinical Psychology Review*, 26, 50–65.

Kelley, S. D., Bickman, L., & Norwood, E. (2010). Evidence-based treatments and common factors in youth psychotherapy. In B. L. Duncan, S. D. Miller, B. E. Wampold, & M. A. Hubble (Eds.), *The heart and soul of change: Delivering what works in therapy* (2nd ed., pp. 325–355). Washington, DC: American Psychological Association.

Kennard, B. D., Clarke, G. N., Weersing, V. R., Asarnow, J. R., Shamseddeen, W., Porta, G., & Brent, D. A. (2009). Effective components of TORDIA cognitive-behavioral therapy for adolescent depression: Preliminary findings. *Journal of Consulting and Clinical Psychology*, 77, 1033–1041.

Kennedy, E., & Midgley, N. (Eds.). (2007). *Process and outcome research in child, adolescent and parent–infant psychotherapy: A thematic review*. London: NHS London.

Kiselica, M. S., Baker, S. B., Thomas, R. N., & Reedy, S. (1994). Effects of stress inoculation training on anxiety, stress, and academic performance among adolescents. *Journal of Counselling Psychology*, 41, 335–342.

Langer, D., McLeod, B. D., & Weisz, J. R. (2011). Do treatment manuals undermine youth–therapist alliance in community clinical practice? *Journal of Consulting and Clinical Psychology*, 79, 427–432.

Lempen, O., & Midgley, N. (2006). Exploring the role of children's dreams in psychoanalytic practice today: A pilot study. *Psychoanalytic Study of the Child*, 61, 228–253.

Leudar, I., Sharrock, W., Truckle, S., Colombino, T., Hayes, J., & Booth, K. (2008). Conversation of emotions: On transforming play into psychoanalytic psychotherapy. In A. Perakyla, C. Antaki, S. Vehvilanen, & I. Leudar (Eds.), *Conversation analysis and psychotherapy* (pp. 152–172). Cambridge: Cambridge University Press.

Linden, W. (1973). Practicing of meditation by school children and their levels of field dependence-independence, test anxiety, and reading achievement. *Journal of Consulting and Clinical Psychology*, 41, 139–143.

Luzzi, A. M., Bardi, D., Ramos, L., & Slapak, S. (2015). A study of process in psychoanalytic psychotherapy with children: The development of a method. *Research in Psychotherapy: Psychopathology, Process and Outcome*, 18, 72–81.

MacKay, B., Gold, M., & Gold, E. (1987). A pilot study in drama therapy with adolescent girls who have been sexually abused. *The Arts in Psychotherapy*, 14, 77–84.

McCauley, E., Gudmundsen, G., Schloredt, K., Martell, C., Rhew, I., Hubley, S., & Dimidjian, S. (2015). The adolescent behavioral activation program: Adapting behavioral activation as a treatment for depression in adolescence. *Journal of Clinical Child and Adolescent Psychology*, 45, 291–304.

McCrea, K. T. (2014). 'How does that itsy bitsy spider do it ?': Severely traumatized children's development of resilience in psychotherapy. *Journal of Infant, Child, and Adolescent Psychotherapy*, 13, 89–109.

McLeod, B. D., Jensen-Doss, A., Tully, C. B., Southam-Gerow, M. A., Weisz, J. R., & Kendall, P. C. (2016). The role of setting versus treatment type in alliance within youth therapy. *Journal of Consulting and Clinical Psychology*, 84, 453–464.

McNeil-Haber, F. M. (2004). Ethical considerations in the use of nonerotic touch in psychotherapy with children. *Ethics and Behavior*, 14, 123–140.

Midgley, N., & Target, M. (2005). Recollections of being in child psychoanalysis: A qualitative study of a long-term follow-up project. *Psychoanalytic Study of the Child*, 60, 157–177.

Miller, S. D., Hubble, M., & Duncan, B. (2008). Supershrinks: What is the secret of their success? *Psychotherapy in Australia*, 14, 14–22.

Miller, S., Wampold, B., & Varhely, K. (2008). Direct comparisons of treatment modalities for youth disorders: A meta-analysis. *Psychotherapy Research*, 18, 5–14.

Perakyla, A. (2010). Shifting the perspective after the patient's response to an interpretation. *International Journal of Psychoanalysis*, 91, 1363–1384.

Peris, T. S., Compton, S. N., Kendall, P. C., Birmaher, B., Sherrill, J., March, J., & Piacentini, J. (2015). Trajectories of change in youth anxiety during cognitive-behavior therapy. *Journal of Consulting and Clinical Psychology*, 83, 239–252.

Reynolds, W. M., & Coats, K. I. (1986). A comparison of cognitive-behavioral therapy and relaxation training for the treatment of depression in adolescents. *Journal of Consulting and Clinical Psychology*, 54, 653–660.

Reynolds, M. W., Nabors, L., & Quinlan, A. (2000). The effectiveness of art therapy: Does it work? *Art Therapy*, 17, 207–213.

Ritschel, L. A., Ramirez, C. L., Jones, M., & Craighead, W. E. (2011). Behavioral activation for depressed teens: A pilot study. *Cognitive and Behavioral Practice*, 18, 281–299.

Rousseau, C., Benoit, M., Gauthier, M. F., Lacroix, L., Alain, N., Viger Rojas, M., & Bourassa, D. (2007). Classroom drama therapy program for immigrant and refugee adolescents: A pilot study. *Clinical Child Psychology and Psychiatry*, 12, 451–465.

Ruzansky, M. (2007). The analytic setting: The establishment of the therapeutic framework in initial psychoanalytic child psychotherapy sessions. Unpublished master's thesis, Anna Freud Centre and University College London.

Schneider, C., & Jones, E. E. (2004). Child Psychotherapy Q-Set coding manual. Unpublished manuscript. Berkeley: University of California.

Semple, R. J., Lee, J., Rosa, D., & Miller, L. F. (2010). A randomized trial of mindfulness-based cognitive therapy for children: Promoting mindful attention to enhance social-emotional resiliency in children. *Journal of Child and Family Studies*, 19, 218–229.

Semple, R. J., Reid, E. F. G., & Miller, L. F. (2005). Treating anxiety with mindfulness: An open trial of mindfulness training for anxious children. *Journal of Cognitive Psychotherapy*, 19, 387–400.

Siegel, C. L. (1972). Changes in play therapy behaviors over time as a function of differing levels of therapist-offered conditions. *Journal of Clinical Psychology*, 28, 235–236.

Slayton, S. C., D'Archer, J., & Kaplan, F. (2010). Outcome studies on the efficacy of art therapy: A review of findings. *Art Therapy*, 27, 108–118.

Smith, J. J. (2010). Therapist self-disclosure with adolescents: A consensual qualitative research study. Doctoral dissertation, Marquette University. Retrieved from http://epublications.marquette.edu/dissertations_mu/86

Smith, P., Yule, W., Perrin, S., Tranah, T., Dalgleish, T., & Clark, D. M. (2007). Cognitive-behavioral therapy for PTSD in children and adolescents: A preliminary randomized controlled trial. *Journal of the American Academy of Child and Adolescent Psychiatry*, 46, 1051–1061.

Stanton, H. E. (1994). Self-hypnosis: One path to reduced test anxiety. *Contemporary Hypnosis*, 11, 14–18.

Sukhodolsky, D. G., Kassinove, H., & Gorman, B. S. (2004). Cognitive-behavioral therapy for anger in children and adolescents: A meta-analysis. *Aggression and Violent Behavior*, 9, 247–269.

Svensson, L., Larsson, A., & Ost, L. G. (2002). How children experience brief-exposure treatment of specific phobias. *Journal of Clinical Child and Adolescent Psychology, 31, 80–89.*

Trowell, J., Rhode, M., Miles, G., & Sherwood, I. (2003). Childhood depression: Work in progress. *Journal of Child Psychotherapy, 29, 147–170.*

Truax, C. B., Altman, H., Wright, L., & Mitchell, K. M. (1973). Effects of therapeutic conditions in child therapy. *Journal of Clinical Child and Adolescent Psychology, 1, 313–318.*

Ulberg, R., Falkenberg, A. A., Nærdal, T. B., Johannessen, H., Olsen, J. E., Eide, T. K., Hersoug, A. G., & Dahl, H. S. J. (2013). Countertransference feelings when treating teenagers: A psychometric evaluation of the feeling word checklist–24. *American Journal of Psychotherapy, 67, 347–358.*

Veale, D. (2007). Cognitive-behavioural therapy for obsessive-compulsive disorder. *Advances in Psychiatric Treatment, 13, 438–446.*

Wall, R. B. (2005). Tai chi and mindfulness-based stress reduction in a Boston public middle school. *Journal of Pediatric Health Care, 19, 230–237.*

Wehr, S. H., & Kaufman, M. E. (1987). The effects of assertive training on performance in highly anxious adolescents. *Adolescence, 22, 195–205.*

Zack, S. E., Castonguay, L. G., & Boswell, J. F. (2007). Youth working alliance: A core clinical construct in need of empirical maturity. *Harvard Review of Psychiatry, 15, 278–288.*

8

CONCLUSION

NICK MIDGLEY, JACQUELINE HAYES AND MICK COOPER

This chapter discusses

- What the evidence tells us, in summary, about the practice of counselling and psychotherapy with children and young people
- Some of the key questions that still need answering
- How readers can stay updated with the latest research
- Some suggestions for conducting your own research

What do we know so far?

Given the evidence reviewed in this book, there are a number of things about the mental health and wellbeing of children and young people – and therapeutic approaches to improving this – that we can say with some certainty:

- Mental health problems in children and young people are common: around 10 per cent of 5–16 year olds have a measurable difficulty. Among some vulnerable groups, such as children in foster care or in the juvenile detention system, the figures are much higher.
- The most common mental health problems in children and young people are emotional and conduct disorders, with a high prevalence of comorbidity across problems.
- Untreated mental health problems in children and young people can have a lifelong negative impact.
- Mental health problems in children and young people are likely to be caused by multiple factors, including child, family and socio-cultural influences.
- Children's early experiences of care, attachment and trauma can profoundly affect how their brains develop, and can underpin the emergence of mental and physical health problems.
- Overall, therapeutic interventions for children and young people show large positive effects on their mental health and wellbeing, with benefits generally maintained after the end of therapy.

- There are preliminary indications that therapeutic interventions for children and young people are **cost-effective**.
- For children and young people with anxiety disorders, cognitive behavioural therapy (CBT) appears to be an effective intervention.
- For children and young people with depression, there is evidence for the effectiveness of CBT, interpersonal psychotherapy, family therapy and psychodynamic therapy.
- For children with conduct problems, parent training programmes appear to be effective; with family-based approaches for young people.
- Many therapeutic approaches widely used with children and young people, including humanistic and psychodynamic therapies, have not been sufficiently researched.
- A positive therapeutic alliance is associated with good outcomes in child and adolescent therapy.
- Children and young people who are more involved and engaged in therapy tend to have better outcomes.
- Therapists with good skills in relating to children and young people, and in guiding the therapeutic work, tend to have better outcomes. In particular, therapist empathy is related to good outcomes with children and young people.
- The **effectiveness** of therapy with children and young people is also associated with a strong working alliance with caregivers. This is particularly important in preventing early drop out in therapy.
- In terms of specific techniques, there is good evidence for using graded exposure for children and young people experiencing anxiety problems.
- There is good evidence for the benefit of using play with children.

Drawing these findings together, what we can say is that the mental wellbeing of children and young people is a major health issue, and urgently needs addressing. We know that psychological interventions can be of benefit, though some approaches have been evaluated far more than others. This means that, in many cases, there is an absence of evidence, which is not the same as evidence that these other approaches are ineffective. Generally, as with the adult psychotherapy field, the best evidence is for specific techniques or programmes (such as graded exposure) for specific emotional or behavioural problems (such as phobias). Again, this is partly because more research has been carried out focusing on children with specific psychiatric diagnoses, or therapies with a cognitive behavioural focus. However, there is also evidence that relationship factors, and a wider pool of techniques and approaches (such as using play), contribute towards positive therapeutic outcomes.

   It is clear that there are many areas where research evidence is missing, or where research has been designed in ways that make it difficult to draw clear conclusions. What much of this points to is the need for far more evidence about what works with children and young people, and also a better understanding of how or why it works, for whom, in what circumstances. There are still many widely used therapeutic approaches for which evidence remains very limited: where we really do not know if, overall, these practices are helpful (or possibly even harmful). There is also a need to understand much more about the process of therapy, and how it might bring about change in children and young people. With such evidence, we can then go on to develop and improve our interventions.

Keeping yourself updated

If you are interested in trying to keep up to date with the latest findings in the child and adolescent counselling and psychotherapy field, here are some suggestions for what you can do:

- Go to the web pages of the main child counselling and psychotherapy research journals and sign up for email alerts – you will then be emailed details of new research articles every time an issue of the journal comes out. Leading journals in the field include: *Journal of Clinical Child Psychology and Psychiatry*; *Counselling and Psychotherapy Research*; *Journal of Infant, Child and Adolescent Psychotherapy*; *Journal of Counseling Psychology*; *Child and Adolescent Mental Health*; *Psychotherapy Research*; *Child and Family Social Work*; *Journal of Child Psychotherapy*; and *Journal of Clinical Child and Adolescent Psychology.*
- Check out the research pages on the website of the British Association for Counselling and Psychotherapy (BACP) – although these pages cover research about therapy with both adults and children and young people, they have good resources, especially for those wanting to carry out therapy research: www.bacp.co.uk/research/
- When wanting updates about **evidence-based treatments** for specific psychological difficulties, search on the following websites:

  o Cochrane Library (such as for parent–infant psychotherapy or childhood depression): www.cochrane.org/
  o National Institute for Health and Clinical Excellence (NICE) (Mental Health and Behaviour Conditions): www.nice.org.uk/
  o American Psychological Association (Division 12) Empirically Supported Treatments: www.apa.org/divisions/div12/rev_est/

- Keep an eye out for new editions of the 'bibles' of psychotherapy research findings, in particular: *The handbook of psychotherapy and behavior change* (Ed. M. Lambert), *What works for whom? A critical review of treatments for children and adolescents* (Ed. P. Fonagy et al.) and *What works with children, adolescents, and adults? A review of research on the effectiveness of psychotherapy* (A. Carr).
- If you are interested in particular areas or research questions, just try Googling them or search on Google Scholar (http://scholar.google.co.uk/) – chances are, something of interest will come up. If you have access to electronic databases (for instance, through a university library), ISI Web of Knowledge and PsycINFO are two of the best search engines for finding the latest studies.
- There are a range of reports on all aspects of counselling with children and young people in the UK on the Counselling MindEd Scoping Reports, and this is a great starting point for further research in this field: www.bacp.co.uk/ethics/Resources/MindEd.php
- To get updates on recent research findings, you can subscribe to a number of blogs and email newsletters which are written in a style to make the findings from research accessible to a wider readership. Some of our favourites are:

- o Mental Elf – the National Elf Service: www.nationalelfservice.net/mental-health/
- o The British Psychological Society Research Digest: http://digest.bps.org.uk/
- o Children's Mental Health and Psychological Wellbeing eBulletin: www.chimat.org.uk/default.aspx?QN = CHMK9

- If you would like to be able to ask questions and join discussions about child therapy research, you can sign up to the online e-forum for the Child and Family Therapy Research (CaFTR) special interest group, which is part of the Society for Psychotherapy Research. Details about the group and how to join can be found on the special interest group section of the website for the Society for Psychotherapy Research: www.psychotherapyresearch.org

Doing your own research with children and young people

While some of the research discussed in this book comes from studies that require a level of resourcing well beyond the capacity of most practitioners (in particular, **randomized controlled trials**, which can cost millions of pounds to undertake), it is also true to say that 'research can be far simpler and more user-friendly than most therapists realize' (Lebow, 2006: 211). Research and evaluation can give therapists an opportunity to find out more about their practice – for instance, what their clients experience as helpful and unhelpful – and it is also an opportunity for therapists to demonstrate the value of what they do (Lebow, 2006). Through undertaking research and disseminating findings, therapists also have an opportunity to contribute to the wider body of knowledge on the process and outcomes of counselling and psychotherapy.

In terms of what practitioners can do, perhaps the most basic level of research is simply to keep systematic records of their work: for instance, how many clients they see, what their **demographic** backgrounds are, and which of their clients appear to do best (Lebow, 2006). At the next level up, therapists can start to systematically evaluate the effectiveness of their work using outcome evaluation forms, such as the Young Person's Clinical Outcomes in Routine Evaluation measure (YP-CORE). Therapists might also want to evaluate their practice by inviting clients to complete service satisfaction forms; or 'target complaint' forms, which ask children and young people to rate their degree of change on individualized questionnaire items (for an excellent resource where many different **outcome measures** can be downloaded, go to: www.corc.uk.net/resources/measures/). If therapists then pool their data with other practitioners (bearing in mind, of course, issues of confidentiality and ethics), it becomes possible to start developing datasets that can be used to test a specific **hypothesis**: for instance, the general effectiveness of gestalt therapy with children. An excellent support for this is the British Association for Counselling and Psychotherapy's (BACP) Children and Young People's Practice Research Network (www.bacp.co.uk/schools/). This is a group of child counsellors and researchers who are working together to generate evidence for their practice, and seeks to support high-quality research in this field.

And finally . . .

Today, it is becoming increasingly difficult for child therapists to evade the call to become research-informed, but it is our hope that therapists can be so much more than that: 'research-inspired', 'research-invigorated', or 'research-revitalized'. Research findings in child and adolescent counselling and psychotherapy can help counsellors and psychotherapists be the best practitioners that we can be for the children and families we work with, and what better sorts of friends would we want to have around?

Questions for reflection

- How would you summarize, for yourself, what you have learnt about effective therapy with children and young people?
- How do you think that therapy with children and young people brings about change? What do you think are the essential ingredients?
- What research questions in this field are you particularly interested in? How could you find out more?

Reference

Lebow, J. (2006). *Research for the psychotherapist: From science to practice.* New York: Routledge.

GLOSSARY OF RESEARCH TERMS

Allegiance bias Potential bias in outcomes when the researcher has an affiliation, allegiance, vested interest, or belief in one outcome over another (e.g. if the researcher evaluating a particular intervention is also a clinician that practises that particular type of treatment, or the researcher is employed by an organization that has a vested interest in promoting the treatment being studied).

Allocation concealment A technique, such as use of a central telephone randomization service, to ensure that researchers cannot influence (deliberately or not) who will be assigned to which group of a study. This is used to prevent bias.

Analysis of variance A statistical analysis tool that separates the total variability found within a dataset into two components: random and systematic factors. The random factors do not have any statistical influence on the given dataset, while the systematic factors do. The statistic calculated by this test is *F*.

Attrition A research phenomenon in which a group gets smaller in number because of members dropping out. The reliability of a research study can be threatened because the people involved drop out for various reasons ('attrition bias', e.g. people who are not improving are more likely to drop out of treatment and evaluation). When people drop out of a study, the results are limited to a smaller and possibly less diverse sample.

Block randomization An approach to randomization in which allocation is made in blocks in order to keep the sizes of treatment groups similar. (See 'stratification'.)

Blinding In research studies where there are two different groups (e.g. ones who received treatment X and another who received treatment Y), those collecting and analysing the data do not know who is in which group. The aim of doing this is to reduce potential bias. A 'double blind' study is one where the people giving the treatment and those receiving it, as well as the researchers doing the outcome assessments, are unaware of which group the participants are in. This is easier to do with drug trials (where a doctor may not know if they are giving a medicine or placebo) than it is in a psychotherapy trial, where it is hard for a therapist not to know what kind of therapy they are offering.

Causal inference The method of inferring that there is a causal relationship between two variables.

Causal relationships Relationship between two things in which one event is the result or effect of another occurring. For example, when a study finds that young people who rate the therapeutic alliance are more likely to drop out of therapy, it is important to discover whether one thing causes the other (a causal relationship), or whether the connection between them is simply chance, or possibly both are the consequence of something entirely different.

Clinically significant change Shifts in outcomes scores that are meaningful (e.g. from scores that are typical for clinical populations to scores that are more typical of non-clinical populations). This can be calculated in different ways, usually based on population norms for that measure (the most obvious is looking at patients who score above clinical cut-offs at one time point, but after an intervention score below the cut-off).

Common factors Those active ingredients that are not associated with just one, or a collection of schools of therapy – examples of common factors might be the therapeutic alliance, or the child's readiness to change.

Control group A group of participants in a research study who are similar to the intervention group in many characteristics (such as age or presenting problem) but not receiving the intervention being studied, or receiving a different intervention, so they can be used as a comparison group to evaluate the effects of the intervention. For example, when evaluating the effectiveness of therapy for children with anxiety, a control group of children might be offered an unstructured play session instead.

Controlled studies A study in which researchers determine which of their subjects receive the factor that is being tested for having a causal influence upon another factor. Those given the hypothesized causal factor make up the experimental group, while those who do not receive such treatment belong in the control group. Ideally, both groups will be balanced with respect to the subjects' various other characteristics. Often this is achieved simply by randomly assigning subjects to experimental or control groups. (See 'observational study'.)

Confounded or confounding variable This is an additional variable which may have an effect on the dependent variable, other than the independent variable. For example, when children in therapy become less depressed (the dependent variable) when seeing a therapist who self-discloses more (the independent variable), that may just be because those therapists are more at ease with themselves generally (the confounding variable).

Correlation The degree of statistical association between two variables, ranging from 1 (total positive association) to –1 (total negative association), with 0 indicating no relationship between the two variables. When two things are correlated that does not necessarily mean there is a causal relationship.

Correlational studies These studies infer a relationship between two variables based on the fact that they occur together, but usually we cannot assume that one caused the other. For example, some adolescents may feel less depressed when they take a placebo pill (a correlation), but that does not necessarily mean that the placebo was responsible for the change in mood.

Cross-sectional studies   Observational studies that involve studying an outcome within a population at a single time point. For example, asking all children on a single day about their level of anxiety would give a 'snapshot' of the rate of anxiety among children at a particular time.

Cost-effectiveness analysis   The technique compares the relative costs to the outcomes (effects) of two or more courses of action. For example, in an outcome study two types of therapy may have similar clinical outcomes, but the children who received one of them may need far more subsequent hospital appointments, and the treatment itself may be far more expensive, making it less cost-effective.

Curvilinear relationship   This describes a relationship between two variables in which up to a certain point, as one variable increases or decreases, so does the other. After this, as one variable increases, the other decreases (i.e. an upturned-U shape on a graph). For example, as stress increases, so does our concentration. But above a certain level of stress, our concentration will decrease. This can also be in the reverse, i.e. as one variable increases, the other decreases up to a point; after this they both increase together (i.e. a U shape on a graph).

Demographic variables   Those variables which concern people's personal characteristics, such as gender, age or occupation.

Dependent variable   The outcome measured (as compared to the independent variable, see below).

Ecological validity   The direct relevance and correspondence of a research study to 'real life'. For example findings from a study using referred patients may have better ecological validity than one using patients recruited especially for the research, as it matches the world of clinical practice more closely.

Effect size   The magnitude of a finding, independent of sample size. In reporting and interpreting studies, both the substantive significance (effect size) and statistical significance (p-value) are essential results to be reported. The most common measures of effect size for outcomes is Cohen's d, which is the amount of difference between two means in relation to the general 'spread' of the data. The rule of thumb to interpret Cohen's d is: $d = 0.2$ (small effect), $d = 0.5$ (medium effect), $d = 0.8$ (large effect). Effect sizes are also often expressed as the degree of correlation (i.e. association) between two variables, or r. Here, an r of 0.1 can generally be considered small, 0.3 = medium, and 0.5 = large. However there is no simple metric which captures the strength of evidence, and we concur with Fonagy et al. that 'a single phrase or number reflects poorly the complexity of evidence' (2015: 20)[1].

Effectiveness   The extent to which planned outcomes, goals, or objectives are achieved as a result of an activity, strategy, intervention or initiative intended to

---

[1]Fonagy, P., Cottrell, D., Phillips, J., Bevington, D., Glasser, D., & Allison, E. (2015). *What works for whom? A critical review of treatments for children and adolescence* (2nd ed.). New York: Guilford Press.

achieve the desired effect, under ordinary circumstances (not controlled circumstances such as in a laboratory). It answers the question: Does this work?

Efficacy   The extent to which a specific intervention, procedure, or service produces the desired effect, under *ideal conditions* (e.g. a controlled environment or lab circumstances). It answers the question: Can this work?

Empirical   Knowledge that is acquired through observation rather than through theory.

Empirically supported treatments (ESTs)   Therapies which are considered efficacious based on evidence from at least two randomized controlled trials conducted by independent teams that have demonstrated them to be superior to a pill or psychological placebo or another bona fide treatment. When there is RCT evidence but not from independent studies, these treatments are sometimes referred to as 'probably efficacious treatments'.

Epidemiology   The study of the distribution and determinants of health and disease in populations.

Epigenetic research   The study of how genetic traits are turned on and off by particular experiences.

Experimental evaluation designs   Studies that look at the effects of a single variable (e.g. treatment). In these designs participants are allocated to different conditions (e.g. treatment groups). As far as possible, all conditions other than the variable of interest will remain the same. The major strength of these designs is that there can be more certainty about the effects of the variable of interest. However, the artificial setting of a laboratory experiment may produce unnatural behaviour which can lack ecological validity (i.e. is not true to real life).

Expert opinion   The perception of someone knowledgeable about a subject. See 'hierarchy of evidence'.

External validity   The extent to which the results of a study can be generalized to other situations and to other people. Naturalistic or qualitative studies often have good external validity, because they describe things as they 'really are'; however they can suffer from poorer 'internal validity'.

Evidence-based practice   An approach to patient care that encourages the integration of research knowledge from clinical trials and outcome studies, with clinical judgement and patient values, to inform therapeutic work.

Evidence-based treatment   Any treatment that is backed by rigorous research evidence. (See also 'Empirically supported treatments').

Goal-based outcome measures   A way of recording at the beginning of therapy what the child, parent and/or therapist wants to achieve from therapy, and thereafter tracking progress along the way in accordance with whether or not these goals are being met. It can allow personal goals to be set, rather than using predefined measures, such as a measure of levels of depression or anxiety.

Hierarchy of evidence   A means of grading the strength of evidence, based on the susceptibility of research findings to bias. This approach, which is used by the UK Department of Health's clinical practice guidelines for psychological therapies and counselling, considers evidence from a meta-analysis of randomized controlled trials as the strongest form of evidence, and evidence from expert committee reports or opinions as the weakest level of evidence. Its value is hotly debated.

Hypothesis   A tentative explanation of certain observations or facts, which can then be tested in a research study. For example, when we evaluate the effectiveness of therapy delivered by professionals compared to the same therapy delivered by untrained adults, we might hypothesize that the therapy offered by professionals will be more effective. (Although the hypothesis may not be confirmed by the evidence!)

Idiographic approach   The term comes from the Greek word 'idios' meaning 'own' or 'private'. Researchers interested in this aspect of experience want to discover what makes each of us unique. Most idiographic research, such as clinical case studies, will focus on one person, or a small group of people, and try to understand their unique experience, even if one has to be cautious about how much the findings might apply to other individuals. (See 'nomothetic'.)

Incidence   An epidemiological measure that relates to new occurrences, for example, how many children develop mental health problems? This might be measured across childhood, or over a set period of time such as across the course of one year.

Independent variable   A variable manipulated by the researcher, while the dependent variable is the outcome measured. For example, when evaluating the comparative effectiveness of two types of therapy for children with obsessions, the kind of therapy offered may be the independent variable, and the reduction in obsessive symptoms would be the dependent variable.

Intent-to-treat analysis   A method of analysis for RCTs in which all patients randomly assigned to one of the treatments are analysed together, regardless of whether or not they completed or received that treatment. This is to avoid bias from 'crossover' and 'drop outs' from the trial. It is thought to more accurately reflect real practice. For example, in psychotherapy research, an intervention may not be successful in engaging many people in the therapy for several reasons (inflexibility, too far to travel, too much time commitment, not being culturally sensitive, poor protocol for engaging clients, etc.). If you only looked at the results for the small number of people who did engage in the treatment (who are likely to be very different from those who did not engage), your findings would not reflect the reality for the treatment as a whole.

Interaction effects   Where the effect of one factor on the dependent variable differs based on levels of another (third) factor. In evaluation research where there are two groups being compared over time (e.g. looking at outcomes over time between a group receiving an intervention and a control group) we are often interested in looking at the interaction of group × time, i.e. do people in each group change in different ways over time?

Internal validity   A property of scientific studies which reflects the extent to which a causal conclusion based on a study is warranted. Such warrant is constituted by the extent to which a study minimizes systematic error (or 'bias'). More controlled studies, such as randomized controlled studies, often have good internal validity, but may have poorer external validity.

Intraclass correlation coefficients (ICC)   A measure of reliability of measurements or ratings (e.g. when data are coded, a subset should be coded by more than one person to check that they are coding reliably, i.e. they agree on their ratings).

Linear relationship   A relationship in which the increase or decrease of one variable corresponds to an increase or decrease in another variable. Graphically this is represented as a straight line.

Longitudinal studies   Observational studies that follow up groups of participants over a period of time.

Mediating variable   The variable that explains the relationship between the dependent variable and the independent variable. For example, children with conduct disorder may have poorer outcomes than children with depression; but on further investigation, it may be that the difference between the two groups is explained by another factor, i.e. that those with conduct problems are more likely to drop out of therapy (the mediating variable), and that this factor explains the difference between the two groups.

Meta-analysis   A statistical procedure which pools findings from different studies to estimate overall effects. It is sometimes considered the 'strongest' form of evidence (see 'hierarchy of evidence') because it is based on the findings of several individual studies, and the findings of each are brought together in a systematic and rigorous manner.

Naturalistic evaluation design   Studies that map out changes occurring in the context in which they occur. There are no changes or manipulations made to usual practice (e.g. interventions and participants). Because there is very little/no interference with the natural environment of the subject, these types of studies are said to be high in 'ecological validity' (true to real life) and, most likely, 'external validity' (findings can be generalized to other real life settings). However the lack of control can make replication very difficult, and allows for a multitude of 'confounding variables' to be introduced.

Nomothetic approach   The term comes from the Greek word 'nomos' meaning 'law'. Researchers who adopt this approach are mainly concerned with studying what we share with others, and thereby establishing laws or generalizations. Most outcome studies are nomothetic, insofar as they compare the outcomes of two groups, rather than exploring individual outcomes. (See 'idiographic approach'.)

Non-experimental studies   Research where the researcher is not manipulating the intervention or controlling who receives it, therefore a cause and effect relationship cannot be proved. These include correlational studies, surveys and case studies.

Non-randomized controlled trial   Studies that are similar in design to randomized controlled trials (see definition below), but in which no effort is made to ensure random (and therefore approximately equal) allocation across groups. For example, a group from one school or geographical location might receive CBT whereas another area might receive person-centred counselling. As a result it is difficult to be sure any difference between the two groups is due to the intervention and not due to differences between children in the two settings.

Observational study   In contrast to randomized controlled trials, these are studies where researchers do not try to manipulate whether their subjects receive the treatment being investigated in the way intended, or randomly allocate participants to different treatments. Observational studies thus are subject to worries about 'confounding' variables, but can have good external validity.

Outcome measures   Measures that are used to determine the results of a study. In child therapy research, outcome measures might be based on questionnaires or on a test, and they can be self-report, or filled in by someone else (e.g. a parent) or based on observation (e.g. a researcher rating capacity to play based on observing a child playing).

Outcome studies   Studies that look at the result of providing a therapeutic intervention, but without a comparison to a group not receiving the therapy.

Paired-sample *t*-tests   A statistical test used to determine whether there is a significant difference between the average values of the same measurement made under two different conditions (e.g. pre- and post-treatment). Both measurements are made on each unit (person) in a sample, and the test is based on the paired differences between these two values. The statistic calculated by this test is *t*.

Power calculations   Statistical calculation used to estimate the sample size required to detect an effect (if there is one) on the outcome variables, with a given degree of confidence. For example, many randomized controlled trials of psychotherapy have relatively small sample sizes, which makes it hard to be confident that an effect has been established, even when the outcomes look promising.

Practice-based research   The systematic collection of information about particular therapeutic approaches or methods (i.e. the use of outcome measures) within real world settings.

Pragmatic trials   Forms of randomized controlled trials (see definition below) which measure the effectiveness of a treatment in situations identical to, or similar to, the conditions of 'real' clinical practice.

Pre-post design   A study where participants are studied before and after the experimental manipulation, but without participants being randomly assigned. For example, a study in which measures of depression are used before and after treatment, without any random allocation to different treatment groups, would be a pre-post design. Although it can demonstrate whether change took place, it makes it harder to establish whether the change was due to the particular intervention, or other factors.

Prevalence   An epidemiological measure that relates to existing occurrences, for example what proportion of children have a mental health problem at any given point ('point prevalence').

Prospective design   A study in which the evaluation design is in place before data collection begins. The main advantage is that decisions can be made in advance about the type of data to collect (and can therefore take into account potential confounding variables), how to collect the data and how to record them. The main disadvantages are that this design is much more costly and time-consuming, and that responses may be biased if participants know they are participating in research (known as the 'Hawthorne effect').

Qualitative meta-synthesis   An approach to integrating results from a number of different but interrelated qualitative studies. Various such approaches have been developed, so that the cumulative findings from a range of related studies may be brought together in a systematic way. The technique has an interpretive, rather than aggregating, intent, in contrast to meta-analysis of quantitative studies.

Qualitative research   Research based on language and which does not use numbers or statistics. This approach is often used to study a topic in depth, and usually aims for meaningful understanding of a phenomenon rather than seeking statistical patterns. Examples include analysing recorded sessions of therapy or asking children and therapists for their views on a topic.

Quantitative research   An approach to conducting research that emphasizes measurement and the statistical, mathematical, or numerical analysis of data often collected through polls, questionnaires or surveys.

Random allocation/Randomization   The process of assigning research participants to treatment or control conditions by chance, to minimize the likelihood of systematic differences between groups.

Randomized controlled trial/Randomized clinical trial (RCT)   An experimental study in which participants are randomly assigned to two or more groups, such that the efficacy of the different interventions can be identified.

Regression to the mean   Statistical phenomenon in which, if a variable is extreme on its first measurement, it will tend to be closer to the average on its second measurement – and, paradoxically, if it is extreme on its second measurement, it will tend to have been closer to the average on its first. Regression to the mean is the major problem with interpreting the results of uncontrolled studies in clinical populations.

Reliable change   An indicator of whether people changed sufficiently that the change is unlikely to be due to simple measurement unreliability. Researchers can determine who has changed reliably by seeing if the difference between the follow-up and initial scores is more than a certain level. There are different ways of calculating this.

Research   A systematic process of enquiry that leads (hopefully) to the development of new knowledge.

Retrospective design   Makes use of previously collected data. The main advantages are that this design is less time-consuming, requires fewer resources, and can often collate larger amounts of data than if a prospective design is used. The main disadvantages are that data may not have been collected and recorded systematically, and important variables may not have been collected.

Routine outcome measures   Session-by-session measures, collecting data that can be used to assess the effectiveness of a treatment.

Sample size   The number of individual pieces of data collected in a study. In most quantitative research, the sample size is important in determining the accuracy and reliability of a study's findings, with a larger sample increasing the chance that the findings may be statistically significant. A 'power calculation' may be used to help decide the best sample size in some studies. In qualitative research, sample sizes tend to be smaller, as there is more of a focus on in-depth exploration and understanding.

Semi-structured interviews   A type of interview in which areas of discussion are planned in advance; however there is scope for the interviewer to explore topics that emerge during the interview in greater detail.

Standardized assessment   An assessment tool that has been designed to measure a child's abilities compared to other children of his or her age. Usually these assessment measures (e.g. IQ tests) have been administered to thousands of children of varying abilities to determine the average level of ability. By contrast, a non-standardized assessment is an informal assessment that therapists or researchers might conduct to determine a child's strengths and abilities, but it is not possible to say how these results might compare to those of other children.

Statistically significant   A research finding that is unlikely to have come about by chance alone. Researchers identify this by setting an acceptable level of risk (typically 1 in 20) and then seeing whether or not the actual data suggest a probability that is less than this (the p-value).

Stratification   A method of allocating participants to two different arms of a study which considers factors other than the type of treatment given. For example, a sample might be stratified according to age, to ensure that a roughly equal number of younger and older children are randomized to two different therapies being compared.

Subject   A person who participates in human subject research by being the target of observation by researchers. Some researchers argue that this language objectifies the people who take part in research, and that they are better described as 'participants' or 'informants'. This shift in terminology can be directly traced to the work of the HIV/AIDS activists and cancer survivor communities in the 1980s and 1990s, who demanded participation in setting research agendas, and felt that the language of experimental psychology could be unhelpful and alienating.

Systematic reviews   A reliable overview of the results of research in one area, using a replicable, scientific and transparent approach. Sometimes these reviews combine the results from a number of studies that have used the same intervention to try and establish an overall effect associated with a particular approach.

Treatment as usual   A condition in which participants receive their usual treatment (which varies between studies), as opposed to the intervention under investigation. Often used as the control in RCTs.

Treatment protocol   A term deriving from medicine which is used to describe a method of treatment to be used in a clinical trial. Also known as 'treatment manual'.

Triangulation   The bringing together of multiple sources of information to form a more detailed picture based on what all these sources are pointing towards. It is a term often used in research when more than one method is used to collect data.

Variable   A characteristic, number, or quantity that increases or decreases over time, or takes different values in different situations. Variables may be categorical (e.g. the ethnicity of a child, which is expressed in words) or quantitative (e.g. a child's age, which is expressed in numbers). In experimental research, there are three categories of variables: dependent, independent and controlled.

Variance   The extent to which the data is spread around the average value. The larger the variance, the more widely the data is distributed.

Wait-list control group   A control group (see above) who are waiting to start an intervention, rather than receiving a different intervention.

INDEX

Printed in Great Britain
by Amazon

64932402R00124